MW00815299

AFTER THE LIGHTS

Find Meaning Beyond College in Five Simple Steps

Mark Steffey

Copyright © 2016 by Mark Steffey

All rights reserved. No part of this publication may be reproduced, distributed, or transmitted in any form or by any means, including photocopying, recording, or other electronic or mechanical methods, without the prior written permission of the publisher, except in the case of brief quotations embodied in critical reviews and certain other noncommercial uses permitted by copyright law. For permission requests, write to the publisher, addressed "Attention: Permissions Coordinator," at the address below.

Mark Steffey
4823 Bayfield Rd
Allison Park, PA 15101
www.afterthelightsbook.com

Printed in the United States of America

Publisher's Cataloging-in-Publication data
Steffey, Mark.
After The Lights: Find meaning beyond college athletics in five simple steps / Mark Steffey

ISBN 978-1539981688
1. Body, Mind & Spirit 2. Inspiration & Personal Growth

Library of Congress #: 2016920848

First Edition

For my wife Kristin

You are the true writer in the family and
the student athlete that I admire most

Contents

Acknowledgements

So many people have been a part of writing this book, and I am certain that without their input, it would have only remained an idea.

The Coalition for Christian Outreach, my employer since 2008, allowed me to a take a three-month Sabbatical to rest and to write. The CCO is the best campus ministry organization out there, and their commitment to the well-being of campus staff is something for which I will always be grateful.

An amazing group of people helped me throughout the various stages of the writing process. I want to especially thank Doug Melder, my aunt Jonellen Heckler, my uncle Lou Heckler, Tyler Wilps, Jon Gratton, my parents George and Nancy Steffey, Kelly Cooke, and Sandi Starr-Everhart. Each of these people took time to help along the way, reading and editing the first drafts of the manuscript and providing valuable input and feedback.

Finally, to my amazing wife Kristin, who is the real writer in the family, for putting up with my constant talking about this project and for encouraging me during every step of the journey.

Author's Note

When writing a book, every author has an important decision to make: fiction or non-fiction. So, I went with neither. And both. Let me explain.

The pages you are about to read are a fictional story. But the story has a direct purpose; to teach five simple action steps. **So as you read the story, my hope is that you use it as a jump start to take action in your own life to make small but meaningful changes for the better.**

The final pages include a summary of the five steps, along with discussion questions that I hope you will find to be helpful. To get the most out of reading the story, you should grab five blank index cards along with a notebook and pen or pencil.

I have included my phone number and email address at the end of the book. I would love to hear from you!

Mark

Introduction

I have spent the past 8+ years, **more than 3,000 days,** among the very best college athletes. In my role as a campus minister/chaplain among Division 1 student-athletes at a "Power 5" state university, I attend practices and games, sit and talk with athletes one on one, meet with them in small groups, take them into the inner city to serve, and lead them to Haiti to work with orphans. **I have been immersed in this world, seeing athletes try to balance the demands of athletics, academics, and social life.**

For the collegiate student athlete, there is an incredible rush that comes from the thrill of competing at an elite level, being rewarded for the intense training and great sacrifices that it took to make it to the pinnacle of their sport.

But then, within four or five years, it's over. For a select few, a professional sports career is the next step in the journey. But as the famous quote and commercial says "There are over 400,000 NCAA student-athletes, and most of us will go pro in something other than sports." The lights fade, and the "real world" beckons. For many, this can be a difficult transition. Away from the structure of the college experience and the feeling of self-worth that they found in sports, many former student athletes struggle, and many are searching for a better way to live.

This easy-to-read story, "fiction with a purpose", will teach readers five simple steps to finding a more meaningful life.

Questions Before Reading

Here are a few questions to ponder before reading this book. Grab a piece of paper or a notebook (and a pen or pencil):

Write down three or four adjectives that describe your life in each of the following areas in the last few months:
- Your Job (vocationally/professionally)

- Physically (fitness and overall lifestyle)

- Relationally –
        friendships:
        dating:
        community involvement:

- Spirituality (faith practices and personal growth)

In each of these areas, would you say you are:
    5   Highly satisfied
    4   Somewhat satisfied
    3   Neutral
    2   Somewhat unsatisfied
    1   Highly unsatisfied

Chapter 1
Monday Morning

Axl Rose's haunting screech and the rhythmic pounding of Slash's guitar riff blared from Zach's phone. The accompanying vibration bounced it off of the bedside table.

"Do you know where you are? You're in the jungle baby...you're gonna die!"

Zach Welton lay face down. His deadweight body strained to move, and slowly his arm reached for the phone to press the screen and stop the sound of the hard rock music. *I need to change that alarm*, he thought. He slowly lifted his head as a small sliver of sunlight came in from the crack in the curtains. *It's Monday*, he realized. Monday always came too soon, and Friday could never come soon enough.

The past weekend had been the typical mixture of drinking, bar-hopping, Uber rides, girls, pizza, and video games. This one was a bit extended, he had to admit, due to the guys having some people over to watch Sunday Night

Football. Recently though, truth be told, he was having a hard time telling a Friday night from a Sunday night or any other night of the week. Last night's game was only background noise to beer pong and flirting. Three beers turned into five, which turned into losing count.

The typical college life, one could say, but Zach wasn't in college anymore. He'd graduated almost exactly one year ago, and his first 12 months in the 'real world' hadn't gone exactly as he had hoped. His Marketing Degree wasn't being put to great use in his job working on a construction road crew, and living so close to campus made him feel like he was a fifth year senior.

While his mind returned to a foggy state of half-sleep, his phone ended its snooze cycle and welcomed him back to the 'jungle' thanks to Guns 'N Roses. This time he summoned enough energy to slide his feet onto the floor, still fully dressed from the night before.

He dragged himself to the bathroom, glancing into the living room on the way. He knew his two roommates, Derek and Chris, were still asleep, and the living room looked like they had both decided to NOT clean up after their little gathering. Empty beer cans and bottles, pizza boxes, and PlayStation game cases littered the floor and coffee table. *Those slobs. I hope they clean it up before I get home.*

Of course, he was just as much to blame as they were. He flipped the bathroom light on, staring at his round face in the mirror, then glancing down at his bloated gut. *Wow, that's getting bigger.* He had this routine down to a science - no shower, but just a quick splash of water on his face, a momentary teeth-brushing, a long effortless stop at the toilet, and he was into the kitchen to grab a slice of cold pizza and head out the door to catch the 12A bus.

It would be a quick 10-minute ride to the City Maintenance building for his 7 am to 3 pm shift. He grabbed his "Southern State" baseball cap from its hook by the front door and slid it over his unkempt head of dirty blonde hair. Same cap he wore throughout his college baseball career – a daily reminder of his glory days.

It was three blocks to the bus stop, and Zach kept his eyes down, his headache pounding almost rhythmically with his steps. Checking the time on his phone, he realized he'd better pick up the pace to avoid missing the bus *again.* The sun was starting to peek up over the three-story apartment buildings on his block, and all was silent on the crisp late March morning. Zach looked down again at his phone. His brisk walk increasing to a slow jog, he glanced toward the end of the block where the bus stopped. It was turning on the opposite corner and would be at his pickup stop in a matter of a few seconds. He quickly transitioned his jog into a sprint, something he had done many times as a ballplayer in college trying to stretch a single into a double. Only now his legs didn't respond exactly as he had hoped. The tightness in his thighs and stiffness of his ankles was shocking, but the weight of his gut is what disturbed him most.

Into a full sprint as the bus came to its stop, Zach was within a few feet of the bus's door, his chest burning from the run. It was only a short sprint, about 50 yards, but it made him realize just how out of shape he had become. Barely climbing on before the bus started rolling forward, he made his way up the three entry steps. He slid his fare into the cash machine. Gone were the days of free bus rides offered to students who carried a college ID. Finding his way to a seat near the front, he slowly slumped back, closing his eyes for a moment and exhaling deeply.

The bus navigated the nearly empty streets through the heart of the Southern State semi-urban campus, dropping off a few people along the way. As it approached the City Maintenance building, Zach stood up and moved to the door to depart. The bus brakes made their low screech, and he waited for the doors to open, then climbed down onto the sidewalk. Walking around to the rear of the building and through the parking lot full of various kinds of construction vehicles, Zach entered the "Employees Only" door and grabbed his timecard off of the board, sliding it through the electronic scanner: *7:04 am.*, read the LED screen. Late again. He realized that he had caught a later bus than the one he needed to take to arrive at work on time.

Striding down the hall towards the staff lounge, Zach stopped and scanned the Assignment Board to see what his work would entail today.

"Federal Street Paving / Flag Man"

Another day of holding a "Stop/Slow" sign? After last night, standing on the side of the street holding a sign was not exactly the way he wanted to spend the next eight hours.

Opening the door to the staff lounge, he was greeted by the other members of the crew with total silence, same as every other day. He nodded to anyone who may have looked up by chance and walked over to the coffee station, pouring himself a bad-tasting cup of caffeine into a small Styrofoam cup. Zach grabbed a bright-yellow fluorescent vest from the row of pegs hanging on the wall and took a seat at one of the plastic chairs that lined the four windowless walls of the small room.

Soon after, the Projects Manager, a tall, thin City Maintenance 'lifer' named Tom, entered the room. Before any of the five men in the room could get to their feet, Tom started in with an abrupt speech,

"Guys, a reminder: this Saturday morning is the mandatory annual community-service requirement for ALL city workers. This year we will packing school supplies at the Community Cares warehouse on 12th Street. Remember, it's *all* city employees, which includes the suits from the mayor's office. I expect everyone to be at the warehouse by 8 am sharp. No exceptions and no excuses. You are expected to stay all morning. It should wrap up by noon."

Tom concluded and stepped outside the door, letting it close behind him.

Slowly, the crew shuffled to their feet and each took a safely helmet from the wall near the door. Zach gulped down the half-cup of coffee that remained in his cup and headed out last. Tom was waiting in the hallway right outside the door. Motioning to his wrist while holding a piece of paper in his other hand, he made eye contact with Zach and sternly grunted, "Late again."

Zach shrugged and slipped his ball cap off his head and into his back pocket, sliding the helmet on and giving Tom a slight cap-tip.

"Zach, this isn't the Southern baseball team and you aren't the star anymore. 7 am means 7 am. This is the last time I warn you."

Just what I need, Zach thought, *getting my ear chewed by Tom for being four minutes late! All this for a measly $12.50 an hour?* Zach realized, however, that it was a job and for now it was the best he could do. "Cs and Ds get degrees" he had told himself in college. He marched through the parking lot with his fellow Paving Crew workers and climbed into the passenger seat of the maintenance truck. *It's only Monday,* he remembered, *four more days of this nonsense until I can let loose again over the weekend.* The time couldn't go by fast enough.

Chapter 2

Friday Night

Where are we headed tonight?
I say we stick with O'Reilly's.
Friday night special on Miller Lite pitchers.

The text appeared on Zach's phone screen as it rested on the couch next to him while he slumped, half-asleep after the long and boring work week. It was from Zach's roommate Chris, who had a *real* job working for a small insurance company, although he seemed to be coasting along and taking his time getting new clients.

That's cool with me.
It's been a long week.

He set the phone down and rose to walk to the kitchen. Opening the refrigerator door, he looked at the bottom shelf and found a depleted stockpile of tall beer cans. Zach grabbed two 20-ounce Bud Lights and returned to his spot on the couch, cracking open one and placing the other on the coffee table in front of him. He enjoyed a long swig, the crisp cold beverage easing his mind as the aroma from the top of the can filled his nostrils.

The taste and smell brought him a sense of familiarity which he had come to know during those charmed days in college. There were many times when the baseball team celebrated a big win with a night of more Bud Lights than anyone could keep count of. They often joked that Bud Light should be their official team sponsor.

Zach remembered those nights as he turned on the 60-inch TV in front of him. He flipped through the channels to find the MLB Network. It had always been a dream of his to play in The Show, and he had gotten closer than many, but as his senior season came to an end the teams just didn't come calling. As a left-handed hitting shortstop, he knew that the young talent coming from the Caribbean was what teams were looking for, and a 5'10", 170-pound college player from a smaller Division One program didn't stand much of a chance of getting noticed. But deep down he knew he had reached his full potential athletically, and it wasn't enough to get him beyond college.

So here he was, throwing down Bud Lights at 5 pm on a Friday while watching baseball "experts" analyze players and break down statistics. It was a far cry from those playing days of only a year earlier, but it was his reality. Before he could ponder any further, he noticed that he had already consumed one of his 20 ounce cans, and cracked open the other. *Might as well get this buzz going early.*

Zach, we are here at O'Reilly's. You coming out?

The next text Zach received was at 9:30 pm, from his other roommate, Derek. Derek was a piece of work. He played two years on the baseball team at Southern State before quitting because he was "tired of being a slave to the athletic department". Derek's view was that college athletes were simply a PR prop for the university and the coaches were only in it for the money. Currently he spent his days as a Barista at a coffee shop and most of his nights playing video games and drinking.

Zach didn't realize that it was already 9:30. He had downed two more beers and had a dizzying buzz going now. He got up and headed outside, grabbing his hat on the way.

When Zach and his roommates were looking for a place to live two years ago after their Junior year, they specifically searched for places in this neighborhood because it was close to O'Reilly's. It had become their "home away from home" and the place where baseball players congregated every Friday and Saturday night. At times it seemed awkward to hang out there now, since most of the crowd were still in college. On the other hand, Zach, Derek, and Chris knew there would always be college girls to talk to and plenty of pitchers of cheap beer to consume. They had jokingly started calling these kind of weekends their "baseball alumni" gatherings.

O'Reilly's was a small establishment, narrow with the bar on the left, a few booths lining the wall on the right, and bathrooms at the back. Three flat screen TVs hung behind the serving area, along with bottles of hard alcohol and neon-glowing beer signs. Zach walked through the front door and looked back to the second-to-last booth, his "boys" regular spot. There they sat, plastic cups in hand, having been joined by three cute girls. He made eye contact with Derek who hollered, "Zach!" and motioned him to the booth.

"Hey, this is Emily, Rachel, and Tiffany," Derek said. "Ladies, this is Zach."

Each girl smiled in turn and raised their semi-clear plastic beer cup. Chris poured Zach two cups from one of the pitchers at the center of the table and handed them to him as he sat down at the end of the booth.

Zach quickly consumed half of one of the cups, and then took the other to his mouth and slugged down the contents with a large gulp.

These days Zach's life consisted of getting through the work week to find some kind of slight satisfaction in the bottom of a bottle, or in this case a plastic cup. Like in his playing days, he considered himself an 'all-in' kind of person. That mentality had served him well as an athlete, which was what brought him to Southern State five years earlier on a full scholarship.

Baseball was his life from the time he was a little kid. The long hours in the batting cage and crisscrossing the country playing AAU as a teen had been rewarded with a chance to play D1. Southern State wasn't his first choice, but it was the only school to offer him a full ride, and he had taken advantage of it, achieving All-Conference Honorable Mention as a Junior and Senior.

Over the next few hours, Zach downed countless cups of beer, losing track by midnight and finding himself slurring his words and stumbling from booth to bar and back. Before he knew what had happened, he was one of the last people left at O'Reilly's. The bartender was closing the taps and clicking off the TVs, "Hey Zach, it's 2 AM. You alright to get home?"

"Uh, yeah, I'm...fine" He mumbled.

Zach shuffled to the door, rubbing his hand across his forehead and adjusting his ball cap, searching his pocket for his phone and apartment key. He stepped out onto the nearly empty street and stared down at his illuminated phone, barely able to make out the group text message that had been waiting for him:

Reminder: be at the warehouse at 8 am sharp for MANDATORY community service   -Tom

He summoned enough brain power to set his phone's alarm for 7:30 am, turning to make the short walk home. As the city streets spun around him, he slowly made his way, swerving along the pavement and navigating the familiar route to his apartment. He fumbled with the keys at the door, nearly falling through it as he managed to get it unlocked, and dragged himself into his room. Within seconds, he passed out, lying on his back with his mouth open and shoes still on.

Chapter 3

Saturday Morning

The bright Saturday morning sunshine was almost more than Zach could handle as he walked through the parking lot full of cars to begin his morning of *mandatory* community service. Last night was a little more drinking than he was even accustomed to, and his body felt like it had been through a brutal off-season workout.

As he approached the front door of the Community Cares warehouse, he rubbed both eyes, attempting to wipe away the headache that pounded across the front of his forehead. Tom, his boss, was waiting at the front door with a clipboard in hand.

"Zach, here *and* on time? It's a miracle!"

He faced the clipboard towards Zach, pointing to his name and handing Zack a pen. He signed his name, barely looking up.

"Let's see," said Tom, "You are in Group 3. Tyler Dunbar's your group lead. You'll be packing notebooks and pencils. Tyler handles PR for the Mayor's office, so try to make a good impression."

Zach pulled open the front door of the warehouse and stepped through the well-lit lobby. He walked through another set of doors and into a large room with rows of storage shelves on the left and an assortment of simple metal tables on the right, each labeled with a numbered sign. Thirty-five or so people were there; a wide variety of City employees, some drinking coffee and others standing near the tables chatting. His eyes searched until he found a table with a sign that read "Group 3" in the far-back right corner.

He moved with his head down, his brain still pounding from his night of drunkenness. He reached to adjust his Southern State baseball cap a little lower over his eyes. He looked up slightly as he approached the table to see a tall, slender man standing there.

"You must be Zach!" welcomed the man, extending his hand with enthusiasm.

Zach sheepishly returned the handshake. *Too much caffeine for this one*, he judged.

"I'm Tyler. Tom told me I'd have a fellow State baseball alum in my group," he commented as he pointed to Zach's Southern State baseball cap. "Class of 2006, 1st baseman. What about you?"

"Uh, I just graduated last spring...2015"

"Awesome," replied Tyler, "Oh yeah, shortstop, right? I came out to a couple of games."

"Right."

Zach did a quick study of Tyler; tall with a short, clean haircut, fit. He looked like he had stepped from the pages of an LL Bean catalog.

"Well," Tyler continued, "great to have another State ballplayer in the group."

Just then a woman approached the table and Tyler greeted her with the same friendliness and joy that he had received moments earlier. Zach stepped away from the table and glanced around the room, noticing that most of the other people shared his lack of enthusiasm for being there. Tyler, however, seemed *more* than happy to be there. He was full of energy and it appeared like he had been awake for hours. *What's up with this guy?* he pondered.

As the morning progressed, the group of City employees used their assembly-line of tables to fill backpacks with an assortment of school supplies - pens, pencils, notepads, binders, folders, erasers, and more. Throughout the time, Zach watched as Tyler warmly engaged each person in Group 3, asking them about their lives and genuinely listening. He calculated that Tyler was around 32 or 33, since he had mentioned that he graduated in 2006. Zach couldn't help but wonder about where *he* would be in 10 years. The prospects didn't look so good. In fact, before that morning he hadn't even thought much about it. He had lived day to day, existing rather than truly living. Instead of *really* living his life, it felt more like life was living him.

The time went by quickly, and soon there was a neatly stacked pile of full backpacks lining the rear wall of the area where they'd been working. As the groups stood near their tables, Tyler walked towards the front of the room, "Hey everyone, can I have your attention for just a minute."

Zach realized that Tyler wasn't only there to help, he was in charge of this event. *Oh yeah,* Zach remembered, *Tom did say that Tyler ran public relations for the mayor.*

"I want to thank you for being here and taking time out of your Saturday morning to help out. I mean, I guess you *had* to be here, but still...thanks. Today, we packed more than 500 backpacks. These will help kids around our city be well-equipped for our 5th annual 'Summer of Learning' extension program. These kids will be more ready for school year in the fall because of this program. I also want to thank the Docherty Family Foundation for funding this program." Tyler motioned with his arm to an older woman standing to the side who had been working at one of the tables. She smiled shyly and nodded to acknowledge him.

"One last order of business," Tyler directed, "a group picture."

People made their way to the rear of the room to stand behind the assembled backpacks. Tyler and Zach ended up standing next to each other as a photographer snapped several shots of the group. When the group started to disperse, Tyler reached out his hand to Zach.

"Great to meet you Zach. Good luck with everything. Go State!"

"Nice to meet you as well," he replied with as much feeling as he could muster.

Chapter 4

Reflecting

Walking home, Zach couldn't help but let his mind wander, mulling over the last year of his life. Meeting someone like Tyler, just a few years older than him, who seemed to have his life together and was full of energy and purpose, made him realize that he was exactly the opposite.

How did he get here? It seemed like just a short time ago he was an eager freshman at State, ready to take on school, baseball and life with vigor. It had been a slow drift throughout his college years...he'd let his grades slip more and more, and, if he was honest with himself, he had to admit that same carefree attitude had affected his baseball effort as well. It wasn't as if he totally checked out. He worked hard at practices, gave a full effort during games, was a good teammate - but did he give his *all* to reach his full potential? Whether it was in season or out of season, his lifestyle choices hadn't exactly been those of someone who was "all in." He ate what he wanted, drank to excess often, didn't rest properly, and wasted endless hours playing video games and just hanging out with Derek and Chris.

During college, he had justified all of it - after all, the demands of being a student-athlete made him feel it was his *right* to relax when he had the chance, to let loose and have some fun. However, Zach started to realize that, a year later, he was still living that way, but *without* baseball in his life. There was something about his morning with Tyler that pointed out to him where he *wasn't* headed in his life, and he didn't like it. But what could he do? With his Marketing degree, his average GPA, and very little experience in anything other than baseball, his future seemed hopeless.

In all honesty, without baseball, he wasn't sure who he was or what life was about. He had placed *all* his eggs in that basket, and it was empty. Zach was empty. These ruminations, rather than leading to a sense of resolve or motivating him to make a change, simply started to give way to despair. He looked down at his body, out of shape, gaining weight seemingly by the day. He sighed deeply, a feeling a general sadness settling over him like a haunting ghost. *Why am I thinking even about this stuff?* He questioned. *This isn't like me.* At that moment his phone vibrated in his pocket,

Hey, where are you?
Thought you'd still be
sleeping after last night.

The text was from Derek.

I had this community service
thing for work. I am almost home.

Cool. Remember, we got tickets
to the Taste of the City thing today.
ALL YOU CAN DRINK! It starts at 4.

They had purchased $40 tickets to an event where you could try samples from the best of the city's food trucks while drinking free beer from some of the area's local breweries. He pushed his earlier thoughts to the back of his mind. *Why focus on this stuff anyway? Better to just let it go. Live and let live. Eat, drink, and be merry, for tomorrow we die.*

Glancing at his watch, he realized he had time for a solid two-hour nap before heading out with the guys for the afternoon and night. Nice, he sighed, Nothing like a little Saturday afternoon siesta.

Chapter 5

Blackout

"Hey! You up?" came the shouting outside of his bedroom door. "It's time to go!"

It was Derek. Zach's body came to life, lying with his ball cap pulled down over his eyes. He tipped the cap up and squinted at his phone, which had been lying on his chest. *3:56 pm.*

"Hey, uh, I have to shower. You guys leaving now?" Zach hollered, still lying on his back.

"Yeah, man, our Uber is here," Derek responded with agitation. "I knocked on your door 20 minutes ago, bro."

"OK, my bad. I will catch you guys there. Where is it again?"

"It's next to our baseball field, 5th Avenue and Greenleaf Street" Derek reminded him.

"Right, right. I'll be there in 30 or so."

"Later," Derek said, his footsteps fading down the hall.

"He's still sleeping," he vaguely heard Derek tell Chris from outside his window as car doors opened and closed.

Zach managed to rise from the bed and headed into to the bathroom for a quick shower and shave. It took him more time to prep for a Friday or Saturday night out than it did to get ready for work. He tried to smile at himself in the bathroom mirror, then laughed at himself for doing such a thing.

Once dressed, he tapped his Uber app on his phone to find a driver within a couple of blocks. He made the request and walked outside to wait. Within minutes a small red Toyota appeared and he climbed in for the short drive to the Taste of the City event. It was a cool afternoon. *Perfect late-March drinking weather,* he thought.

The little red car zipped through the city streets until it reached Zach's destination, letting him out right across from the baseball complex where he had spent countless hours in college. The street was blocked off from traffic with large wooden barriers, and lined on both sides with various food trucks. The crowd meandered amongst the trucks, people eating and drinking and laughing. Zach hopped out of his ride and stopped at the makeshift gate, giving a girl his ticket as she placed a blue paper wristband on his right forearm. "Have fun," she said, as she handed him a large red Solo cup.

Zach found Derek and Chris where he knew they would be; at the Hombres Locos Taco Truck. They each had a beer in one hand and a foil-wrapped messy taco in the other.

"Zach, you've got to try the new draft from Stonehouse Brewery," Chris said, bypassing any normal greeting as he took a large gulp from his cup.

"Nice to see you too bro. Thanks for waiting for me," Zach quipped.

"Chill, dude. We're all here and the beer is flowing," chimed in Derek.

"Amen!" Chris agreed, raising his cup.

Zach turned away from them and to the booth on his left where Stonehouse Brewery was serving a variety of local ales. He handed the booth worker his cup for a filling of the beer his friends had mentioned and returned to their small huddle. They had been joined by four girls, all of whom looked as if they had been drinking since well before the event's start.

Zach and his friends talked with the girls, each trying their best to look and sound interesting. He attempted to stay involved in the conversation, but occasionally his gaze would catch the baseball stadium lights, towering in the background behind the food trucks. He was taken back to all of the time he'd spent over there. *Funny, I am so close to that place, yet so very far away.* He didn't allow those thoughts to linger. A few more drinks all of his stress would fade away.

As the hours went by, the former ballplayers took full advantage of the unlimited supply of beer, downing cup after cup. Zach lost count somewhere around 8 pm, and by 9 pm the event was coming to an end and the crowd began to thin out. He was stone cold drunk. His mind beyond fuzzy, he could barely remember where he was or what he was doing there.

With a half full cup in his hand and his eyes starting to droop, he wandered through the crowd, having lost track of Derek and Chris. He bumped into a person here and there, his drink sloshing in the cup as he took random sips.

Without thinking about it, he had made his way to the far end of the street where people were exiting to walk home or take ride-shares. He took one last gulp and tossed his cup onto an overflowing garbage can.

He stumbled, barely able to stand, and found himself facing the left-field fence of the baseball field. For some reason, he thought that scaling that fence would be a good idea. He didn't comprehend why. Like a burglar on the prowl, he scanned the area to see if anyone was watching, although it wouldn't have mattered if anyone was.

He grabbed the painted-green metal fence and managed to find enough strength to maneuver himself up and over the 7-foot high barrier. Still not completely processing what he was doing, he slung his right leg over the top, then his other leg, before clumsily tumbling over. As he fell, his arms managed to grip the field-side of the fence. He imagined himself as a covert operative from a first-person-shooter video game. He pushed away from the fence and started a slow prowl towards the infield.

The area being dimly lit only by ambient light from the surrounding streets, Zach told himself he was safe and doing something totally normal. His brain felt like a ship at sea, sloshing side to side in his skull as he weaved his way slowly toward home plate.

Arriving there, he veered left to face the pitcher's mound, holding an imaginary bat in his hands as he brought them together and stood in a serious batting stance. He mumbled something to himself about the pitcher and the inning and the runners on base and swung the pretend bat, his body spinning wildly. He fell to the ground as the phantom baseball sailed over the centerfield wall. "Home...run!" he slurred as he collapsed in the dirt.

Laughing at himself and getting to all fours, he pushed up to a half-standing pose and faced the home dugout. His eyes focused upon the spot on the players' bench where he had sat during college. He forced himself to walk there, conjuring all of his concentration to arrive at that exact place.

He stumbled down the dugout steps and walked clumsily to the bench. As he sat down, his hat dislodged from his head and fell to the ground in front of him. He swayed down wildly to pick it up, falling to the earth.

Laughing again, he picked up the cap and held it in front of his face. The words "Southern State" looked at him with a taunting gaze. He laughed again and plopped the cap on his head, pulling himself onto the bench and resting his head back against the cement wall.

He closed his eyes, and within seconds, blackness.

Chapter 6

Wake Up Call

"Zach?"

The low, familiar voice flooded Zach's ears like a rush of cold water. He strained to open his eyes. He managed to lift his eyelids enough to see Mike Emlinger, his old college coach, standing in front of him. *Am I dreaming?* Zach thought.

"Whoa, man. You *stink*," Coach Emlinger squinted his face and backed away from Zach's slumped body that still rested on the dugout bench.

Zach pushed up to a sitting position and rubbed his eyes, clearing his throat and letting out a shallow cough.

"You are in rough shape, Zach. How the heck did you end up in here, anyway? Don't tell me. I can guess."

"Coach, I'm so sorry. I must have come over here after last night...the food truck thing out on the street."

Coach Emlinger stepped away and leaned against the low front wall of the dugout, his body silhouetted against the sun rising over the horizon.

"Let's get you on your feet."

"Really, I'm sorry. Wow, you must think I'm a mess," Zach said.

His coach walked over and grabbed a paper cup from the top of a large cooler, dispensing water from the spout, then handed it to Zach.

"Zach, as soon as I saw you lying here, I pictured myself back when I was a year out of school. I was in low-A minor league ball, spending more time at bars than I was at the ballfield. It was a rough year."

He was surprised to hear the coach talk like that. In his time as a player, he had only heard coach talked about baseball and school, and not much else. He had never genuinely considered that Coach Emlinger was a real person, with a real past and a life away from baseball.

Zach took a drink of water from the cup and slowly got to his feet. Coach Emlinger put his hand on Zach's shoulder and gave him a light squeeze.

"Listen," he advised, "There is a guy who used to play for me here, a few years before you. I would love to put you in touch with him. I mean, if you are interested. Simply someone to talk with, maybe learn a little about life from. He's helped a lot of my former players who were in your...situation."

Zach's head was still slightly foggy, and he ached from head to toe, like he had been run over by a truck. He didn't know what else to say, so he just replied "OK, that's cool."

Coach took his phone out of his pocket and scrolled through his contacts, then pointed the screen at Zach, "This still your number?"

Zach nodded, and he and the coach turned towards the dugout steps.

"Coach," Zach said, "Again, I'm sorry."

"Hey, don't worry about it. Promise me you'll respond when this guy reaches out to you"

"I promise."

Zach ascended the steps and slowly walked, head down, up the third base line and out through the gate in the fence. He could feel coach's eyes on him, but not as much as the heavy shame that rested on his shoulders.

Chapter 7

Contact

After the long trek home, Zach went straight to his room and fell into his bed. He stared blankly up at the ceiling.

What just happened?

What am I doing with my life?

This is not who I am and this is not the path that I want to be headed down.

But how do I make things different?

I wish I could rewind the clock, back to college and those good times.

But he knew that wasn't a possibility. He knew that this *was* his reality; living just steps from campus in the same apartment as in college, and with the same roommates; working at an unfulfilling job; drinking too much; eating like a pig. And without any plan for things to change anytime soon.

He took his phone out of his pocket and opened his photos, scrolling slowly through the album titled "Senior Year" - baseball action shots, goofy moments from the locker room, times with the guys at parties, even some pictures of him and his parents posing happily at Senior Day and at graduation. *Those were the best times of my life. I can't go back. I can't go back?*

As he looked at the phone's screen, a text appeared across the middle...

Hey, is this Zach?

It was from a number he didn't recognize. A girl he talked to last night?

Yes, it is. Who's this?

He tried to recall if he gave his number to anyone, but it was all a blur.

Coach Emlinger gave me your number and said that you would be interested in meeting up sometime.

Zach suddenly remembered that he had given Coach Emlinger permission to give his number to an older State baseball alum. He didn't imagine he'd be hearing from him this soon.

Oh, right.   Yeah, I am up for it.

How about tomorrow.
I play basketball with some
guys after work. You want to join us?
We could chat then.

Zach sat up, placing his legs to the side of his bed and examining his bloated gut.

Yeah, that sounds good.
When and where? I work until 3.

4:30 at the Parkside Rec Center.
42 Center Ave.

Who is this, actually?
So I know who to look for tomorrow.

I will wait for you at the door.

You'll know me when you see me.

Zach's head was spinning, not from intoxication, but from what he'd just agreed to. *I am out of shape, my life's a mess, and I am meeting a total stranger who won't tell me his name to play basketball? This is weird!*

As the texts cleared from his phone, it returned to a screen showing a picture of him standing at graduation, dressed in his black robe with his parents at his side and his diploma under his arm. He reminded himself that after a full year out of school, things were at a dead end. *Maybe a meeting with this guy is what I need,* he considered. *Maybe it's is a chance at a fresh start.*

Turn to page 149 to find Discussion Questions for Chapters 1 through 7.

Chapter 8
Step 1: SWEAT

Zach decided to chill on Sunday night, and easily fell asleep a little before 10 pm. He got up earlier than normal on Monday morning, giving himself time to shower and eat a bowl of cereal before heading to work. He was able to catch an earlier bus, and was waiting for it when it arrived.

Tom, his boss at work, was sarcastically glad to see him arrive "on time for once" and congratulated him for attending the community service event on the previous Saturday.

After a typically boring day at work, Zach arrived home at 3:30, grabbed a quick snack and went to his room, scouring the closet to find his old basketball shoes. Dislodging them from a pile of unorganized footwear, he threw them in a small gym bag along with an extra t-shirt.

He slung the bag over his shoulder and headed outside for the 20-minute walk to meet his "mystery mentor" for an afternoon of basketball. Zach had played in high school and considered himself a pretty good shooter and defender, but he was so out of shape that he was truly nervous about playing.

The city blocks between his apartment and the Parkside Rec Center were busy with people getting out of work and students leaving classes to return to apartments and dorms. This hustle and bustle was one thing he had always loved about being a student at Southern State. He preferred the mixture of the college campus within the busyness of the city.

He started to break a bit of a sweat as he got within a block of the Rec Center. Turning onto Center Avenue, he could see a tall, slender man holding a basketball leaning against the wall of the building near the front door. *This must be the mystery mentor himself.*

As he approached, it occurred to him that he had seen this guy somewhere before recently. The man looked at him as he got within a few steps and warmly greeted him,

"Zach, we meet again!"

It was Tyler, the guy from the community service day at the warehouse!

"Small world, huh!" Tyler exclaimed, sticking out his right hand for a firm handshake.

"Yeah, small world," he replied quizzically.

Tyler continued, "Honestly, I was stunned when Coach called me yesterday morning. He described you and I knew it must be the same Zach who was at the warehouse Saturday morning."

Zach was stunned too. He had just met this energetic guy a couple of days ago, and here they were, about to play basketball and start some kind of strange "mentoring" thing.

"Well, it looks like you are ready to go," Tyler said, motioning to the gym bag hanging from Zach's shoulder, "Let's head in."

Tyler led Zach through the door and signed them in at the front desk. The desk attendant knew Tyler by name and Zach could tell from her smile that she was happy to see him.

They walked along a short hallway to the left and entered the gym. A few guys were already there, sitting on the wooden bleachers, tying their shoelaces and straightening their shorts. Zach was introduced to the group.

"*Another* former State baseball player, Tyler? Does he run up and down the court like a maniac like you?" quipped one of the older guys.

"You're mad cause you can't keep up, Bill!"

Bill laughed and gave Tyler a fake jab to the chest.

Zach sat down and took off his old beat-up running shoes and replaced them with his seldom-used basketball sneakers. He stood up and leaned forward, stretching his legs and working out the tightness in his lower back.

A few more guys trickled into the gym, and after some small-talk and shooting around, they split up into two teams of five, plus a sub each, and began their full court game. Zach kept up with them, his younger age and general athleticism masking his lack of cardio conditioning. Tyler, however, *was* a maniac, chasing down loose balls, grabbing almost every rebound, and playing relentless defense. He rarely shot, but set screens and made smart passes to set up his teammates for easy scores. Zach noticed that Tyler did all of this with a positive, encouraging attitude, all the while being very competitive.

After three games to 11, the guys finished playing and all sat on the short set of bleachers, drinking water and wiping their faces with towels. Tyler seemed to be the leader. He engaged most of them in conversations that indicated that he knew a lot about each of them. He asked about their kids and work, and listened to their words while maintaining eye contact.

After a few minutes, the gym emptied out and Zach and Tyler were left alone together on the bleachers.

"So," Tyler began, "Coach Emlinger didn't tell me a lot and I don't know much other than you graduated last year. And of course that you are working for the City Maintenance Department. What's your story?"

"Uh, I don't really have a story," Zach replied. "I've been out for a year, been working, hanging out. Living life, I guess."

Tyler listened carefully.

"Got it, got it. Living the dream, right?" Tyler said with a hint of sarcasm, "Well, here's the thing. Not too long ago, I was right where you are. I'm only 32, and 22 and 32 aren't as far apart as you might imagine. Time flies. You'll wake up one day and wonder where it all went. When I got out of school, I had hoped to keep playing, but it didn't work out. I found myself here in the city, while most of my teammates had moved on to other places or to grad school." Tyler leaned in and his tone became quite serious.

"It wasn't more than a few months until I realized that I needed to make some changes. College was over. Baseball was over. I had to figure out who I was, what I wanted to be about, and where I wanted to go with my life."

He paused, as if waiting for Zach to speak, then leaned back folded his arms in front of him, his eyes focusing across the gym, as if he were looking through the wall of the building and out into the world.

"Over the last few years I have kept things simple, focusing on a few principles which have helped me become more and more of the man that I desire to be. Five simple ways to change things for the better.

Zach was listening intently. He could definitely use some help. He resonated with what Tyler was saying about his life so far after college, and he knew that he didn't want to continue down the path he was on.

"These few principles, what exactly do you mean? Like yoga or meditation or something?" Zach asked.

Tyler chuckled, "No, not exactly."

Tyler reached into his gym bag and took out a single 4 x 6 index card. He held it facing himself and studied it as if to reading what was written on it. Zach waited.

"For me, it's five simple practices that I keep at the forefront of my life. They serve as guidelines, reminders of what works for me," Tyler sounded casual and calm, like a friend rather than some sort of 'mysterious mentor' or expert.

"Here's the first one," he said, and handed Zach the index card.

Zach read a single word at the top of the blank card:

SWEAT

"Sweat?" Zach asked, assuming that the card would have something far more profound on it.

"Yep. That's it," Tyler explained, "Just Sweat."

Zach tilted his head slightly and drew his eyebrows down in slight confusion. Tyler gave explained further.

"For me, one of the ways I am made, as a person, is that I have to be active. I looked back at my childhood, at my teenage years, and college, and all the way through I noticed that I felt most *myself* during times when I was active. I always loved to play sports. It's what led me to State, and when I graduated, for some reason I assumed it meant I was done, 'retired' - from sports or being active. You guys still call non-athletes NARPS?"

"Yeah, Non Athlete Regular Person," Zach replied with a hint of laughter.

"Right, and I *was* a NARP. But not anymore and not for a long time now. In fact, I am in better shape today than I was 10 years ago. I'm not a tri-athlete or some kind of elite runner, but I have found what works for me. I sweat, almost every day. Today, it's basketball, as well as on Wednesday, and on the days that I don't play hoops I go to gym for an intense group workout, which challenges me to compete with myself, to set and reach goals. I rest on Sundays."

Zach looked down again at the index card, contemplating what Tyler was saying. He too could remember being very active and loving all sports as a kid. He remembered long days of playing outside, travel baseball, high school basketball, and even the enjoyment of off season weight training during college. Granted, he didn't love *every* moment of it, but he loved the way he felt after each session. Like his body was alive and functioning and thriving. Tyler paused for a long time and could tell Zach was processing his words.

"So... you want me to join your gym?" asked Zach.

"No," Tyler smiled, "Not at all! You have to find out what is right for you...running, a gym, kayaking, biking, heck, even yoga!"

Sitting here after an hour of basketball, it occurred to Zach that it did indeed feel good to sweat.

"Before the next time we get together, take the card and write down your two or three 'Sweat' activities. Be simple, specific and smart. Don't overanalyze it," Tyler concluded, standing up from the bleachers and putting his gym bag over his shoulder.

"OK, I can do that," Zach agreed, standing and placing his basketball shoes into his bag.

They turned together to exit the gym, and Tyler initiated the next part of the process,

"This Wednesday night Southern State plays a midweek game at home. Are you able to meet me there? We could watch the game and talk more."

Zach thought ahead to Wednesday, knowing that his weeknight schedule was *always* open.

"Sure, that works," he agreed.

"OK, great, lets meet at the gate at seven. Bring your index card with your Sweat plan."

Chapter 9

Sweat Plan

When Zach returned to his apartment, Derek and Chris were sitting on the couch engrossed in PlayStation, with a pizza in front of them, each with a beer bottle resting on the coffee table. A scene he'd come home to a thousand times.

"Hey Zach, where have you been? We were worried you might have died! Did you get any of my texts?" Derek asked.

"Uh, no, I guess I didn't," Zach took his phone out of his pocket to see unread texts from Derek…

Dude, where are you?

Grab a case on your way home from work, we are running low

Helloooooooo????

"Oh, well, sorry, obviously I didn't grab a case. I was playing hoops with…. with some guys from work," Zach didn't know how to explain his meeting with Tyler.

"Well, these are the last two beers, so if you were planning to drink tonight you are outta luck, unless you plan on going out." Chris piped in.

"No, I'm good," Zach returned.

"Your loss, bro," quipped Derek.

His roommates resumed their game, while Zach walked down the short hallway, dropped his bag in his room, grabbed a towel and headed for the shower.

Once he was cleaned up, he closed the door to his room and sat on his bed, taking the index card from his gym bag and a pen from the drawer of his bedside table.

He read the card with "SWEAT" written at the top of it. *I need to come up with a plan to get in shape, essentially? Let's see…*

He jotted down the word "Jog." He took out his phone and opened his Map App, typing in his address and the address of the City Maintenance building where he worked.

3.3 miles

Not too far, he thought. *I will have to get up a bit earlier before work. That sucks.* Under the word "Jog", he wrote "to work; Monday, Wednesday, Friday" remembering Tyler said the steps needed to be <u>simple</u>, <u>specific</u> and <u>smart</u>. A little over three miles, three days a week; that seemed manageable.

SWEAT

Jog, 3.3 miles: Monday, Wednesday, Friday – for four weeks

He wasn't sure what to write next, if anything. He wrote down more about the jogging, "for four weeks"

OK, Zach concluded, that seemed doable. Since it was Monday, he knew he could take the bus tomorrow.

He wondered if Tyler was expecting more. He deliberated for another minute, then decided to write again,

"Starting May 1, Join a gym and lift weights Tuesday and Thursday after work for 45 minutes."

SWEAT

Jog, 3.3 miles:
Monday, Wednesday, Friday
– for four weeks

Starting May 1, Join a gym and lift weights Tuesday and Thursday after work for 45 minutes.

He reviewed his plan and knew it was something that he could manage; <u>simple</u>, <u>specific</u> and <u>smart.</u>

He read over the card with a sense of satisfaction and placed it next to his bedside table.

Looks like I am about to Sweat, Zach laughed to himself.

Chapter 10

Breaking A Sweat

Wednesday morning, Zach's alarm sounded at 6 am. He'd taken extra jeans, his work shirt and boots with him to the maintenance building on Tuesday and left them in the staff lounge. This motivated him to get up and exercise. It was a way of keeping his plan simple, specific and smart.

He dressed himself in his old State standard-issue sweatpants and hoodie, and tied on his old running shoes, sighing to himself, knowing that he wasn't exactly looking forward to this three mile run. At the same time, it made him remember early morning workouts with the baseball team. While he dreaded getting up, once he got his blood flowing he thoroughly enjoyed it. He hoped that would be the case today.

He walked out to the curb, pausing to do a few stretches to loosen up his legs. He started off slowly, jogging along the sidewalk, feeling the crisp spring air against his face and breathing it into his lungs. He kept a steady, easy pace as he made the route towards work.

Soon enough, he did feel himself start to sweat, as his heart rate increased, and his mind started to clear. He'd experienced this feeling many times before on long conditioning runs, and it was a sensation he'd almost forgotten. It was like the exercise was clearing his mind of clutter and stress. He started reflecting about life, about what he'd already learned from Tyler and what he might learn next. Time went by quickly and before he knew it he was at the City Maintenance building. He peeked at his watch to see the time: 6:50 am. He was *early*.

Chapter 11

Step 2: STOP

After another day flipping a "Stop / Slow" sign while the patching crew fixed potholes left over from the winter, Zach took the bus home from work, watching out the window almost the whole way and recalling his route from the morning. A sense of satisfaction came over him. *I did it*, he reflected, *I got started with my Sweat plan.* He gave himself a mental pat on the back.

Still good for 7?

The text from Tyler appeared.

Yes, see you there.

Zach entered his apartment to find Derek in the living room, planted in his usual spot on the couch,

PlayStation controller in hand, with a bottle of beer and a half-eaten box of cold pizza in front of him. Several other empty beer bottles littered the table. He was in sweatpants and a t-shirt.

"No work today?" Zach questioned.

"Nah. Well, I, uh, sort of got fired." Derek replied casually.

"Fired? For what?"

Derek didn't look up from his game, "The manager said I wasn't bringing the right 'positive attitude' to the job, that I was 'hurting the coffee culture' or some BS. I hated that job anyway."

"So what are you going to do?"

"No idea, but for now I am going to sit here, get wasted, and kill some zombies," Derek twisted the game controller sideways, furiously pressing buttons.

"Well, good luck," Zach said.

He headed to his room, went in and shut the door behind him. He plopped down on his bed and landed his head on the stack of three pillows at the top, then reached to his bedside table and grabbed the index card, scanning at his "Sweat" plan again. *Well,* he thought, *at least I started. Gotta start somewhere, right?*

After a quick shower, he got dressed, slid the index card into his back pocket, and headed out to make the walk to the baseball game to meet Tyler. It was a long journey, but he didn't mind. It was a cool, sunny spring evening; perfect weather for a ballgame.

He grabbed his go-to sub at Subway, the Spicy Italian, and ate it as he walked through the campus streets.

As he approached the home plate gate, he saw Tyler leaning against the brick facade of the stadium. Zach knew what was coming next -- a firm, friendly handshake and a warm greeting.

They made their way into the mostly empty stadium, where a scattering of parents and college kids dotted the 20-or-so rows of the seating area that surrounded the infield. Tyler led them to a couple of seats about halfway up the first base line, and they sat down just as the Southern State team took the field for the top of the 1st.

"This kid on the mound is a beast," Tyler commented as they settled in.

"You don't have to remind me," Zach said, "He was tough to hit in our inter-squads. Pretty nice to have a midweek starter who can throw that kind of stuff."

The game started, and Tyler jumped right in, "How's your Sweat Plan coming along?"

"Believe it or not, it's going well. I mean, I started today, but I started," Zach said as he leaned forward and took the index card out of his pocket.

He handed it to Tyler. Tyler read the card to himself:

SWEAT

Jog, 3.3 mile:
Monday, Wednesday, Friday
– for four weeks

Starting May 1, Join a gym and lift weights Tuesday and Thursday after work for 45 minutes.

"You ran today?" he quizzed.

"Yep. Got up early. It was a little bit of a struggle, but I made it."

"Great," he handed the card back to Zach, "This is the exact kind of simple, specific, and smart plan that I was talking about. You'll be able to track it, and I like how you gave yourself a month of running before you added another activity. Something to build towards."

Zach put the card in his pocket. Their attention turned to the field, as a visiting player hit a high pop-up into foul territory behind first base, just in front of them. The lanky left-handed first baseman camped under it, a few feet from the protective netting, and called off the pitcher, making the catch a few feet from the visitors' dugout.

"Told you, this guy has filthy stuff. Only eight pitches to get three outs," Zach commented.

Tyler nodded his head, "Yeah, he struck out the second guy on three straight cutters. Painted the zone."

The two sat silently as the teams warmed up for the next half-inning.

Zach piped up, "What's next? I mean, not in the game, but what's next in this, uh, you know, for me?"

Tyler laughed, "I love the enthusiasm. Here is the next simple step to take."

He reached into his pocket and pulled out the next index card. He handed it to Zach and watched him read the word written on the top of it:

STOP

Just then, the Southern State leadoff hitter ripped a sharp line drive in front of them. It landed in fair territory behind the first base bag and zipped along the outfield grass and into the right field corner. The speedy player rounded first and headed for second, looking to the third base coach to see if he should go for a triple. The ball took a funky carom off the base of the wall and bounced past the right fielder. The third base coach motioned for the runner to keep going, as if he might wave him home for an attempt at an inside-the-park homerun, but the right fielder recovered, barehanded the ball and in one motion made a strong line drive throw to the cutoff. As the player was about to round third, the third base coach changed his sign, holding up both hands and signaling for him to stop at third. The player quickly slammed on the brakes as he came to the bag for a stand-up triple.

"OK, 2-4!" "Way to get us started, 2-4!" Came the cheers from the State dugout.

Tyler looked at the card that was now in Zach's hands, "Ha, perfect timing. STOP." he joked.

What, exactly, did this STOP card mean? He wondered.

Tyler read his thoughts, "Stop means stop. It means to take stock of your life and decide to cut out things that are holding you back. Things that are getting in the way. Bad habits, bad choices. Anything you recognize is stopping you from progress. Some things may be addictions."

"I just need to stop? That's it?"

Tyler shook his head in agreement, "That's it. Many people live in fear. Fear of giving up the stuff in their life that they are comfortable with, but some of those things are slowly killing them. The world hates a quitter. But quitting the stuff in life that holds us back, nothing could be wiser."

Zach immediately had a few parts of his life come to mind, but knew that those things were what he was accustomed to. Quitting them wouldn't be easy.

Tyler continued, "When I got out of school, the number one thing I had to quit was a relationship. Can you believe it? I had dated this girl for three years, but we weren't right for each other. When you are with someone that long, it seems like staying together is easier. She was a good person, don't get me wrong, but we both knew it wasn't going to last. Putting a 'stop' on the relationship was tough. It was also the right choice for both of us."

Zach's attention turned to the field, where a State batter had hit a soft liner over the second base bag, scoring the runner from third.

"See what happened there, Zach? Perfect, perfect. Number 24 was able to score only because he stopped after hitting that triple down the line. Stopping is what enabled him to go when the right time came, in this case when the next batter hit him home. Life is like that. You can't go where you want unless you stop when you should."

"What should I stop?" Zach asked.

"It's up to you. But like Sweat, keep it simple and specific. Don't overthink it. Discern what those things are that you have to cut out. It might only be one thing. It might be two or three."

Zach took the index card and slid it into his pocket alongside his Sweat card.

"OK, when is this assignment due, professor?" Zach joked.

"Professor, huh? That's a first! I am glad you asked. You know the ballfield over on Evergreen Street?"

"Sure," Zach replied, picturing it in the neighborhood south of the campus.

"Well, do you have time to meet me there Saturday morning at 10?" Tyler said.

"Yes, I can do that."

"Great, wear athletic clothes and bring your glove," Tyler instructed.

They sat together for the next few innings, watching and talking, mainly about the game. Zach liked that their time together wasn't *all* serious. Tyler seemed interested in more than "telling Zach what to do." Whether it was the basketball game they played or this baseball game, their time together was mainly spent casually. Tyler seemed to care more about being present than about dispensing life-changing knowledge.

As the evening darkened into night, the stadium's lights illuminated the field. The game came to a close; a solid 6-1 State victory. Zach and Tyler got up and made their way to the home plate area exit, shaking hands as they departed.

"See you on Saturday morning, Zach. Bring your STOP plan," Tyler said with a smile as they headed their separate ways.

Chapter 12

Stop Start

The next morning Zach got up a little earlier than normal for work, even though it was Thursday and not one of his running mornings. He made himself a cup of coffee and headed to the living room with his "STOP" index card in hand.

He relaxed on the couch, made some space on the cluttered table in front of him, and sipped from his hot mug. He cleared his mind and contemplated what he would write on the card.

He glanced at the TV screen, then down at the PlayStation console that rested on the base of the TV stand. It was his PlayStation. He had purchased it a couple of years ago after saving up some money from his stipend checks. He had played it way too much over those years, and he knew he wasted lots of time playing video games even now. It occurred to him that perhaps this could be one of his "Stop"s.

A handful of the games belonged to him as well, as did the four game controllers. Probably worth about $500 if he listed it on Craigslist.

Why not now? He supposed, getting up from the couch. He arranged the console, controllers, and games in a nice display, and took a picture with his phone.

He went onto the mobile Craigslist website, and after a few clicks, the console was listed for sale.

He returned to the couch and wrote on the index card:

STOP

Video Games

OK, that's one thing. What's next?

He remembered what Tyler had said about not being able to "Go" until you learn when and what to "Stop." It was clear as day. Zach knew what was next on the list, and he knew it would be a drastic, difficult change. He needed to stop drinking. Not stop drinking *so much*, just stop altogether. That notion disturbed him. He started reminiscing about college. Rarely had there been a time since early in his freshman year when he had gone *a couple of days* without imbibing. He had always assured himself that alcohol wasn't a problem for him, but as he made a 'sober' assessment, he had to admit that he drank often and usually more than he had intended. It was only a few days ago that he found himself passed out in the baseball dugout.

But to stop? Could he really stop drinking, straight up? He wasn't sure. But he was sure that he didn't like where he was in his life. He lived for the weekend. He lived for the release and escape that came from being drunk. And he knew that was no way to live, to truly live.

With a bold press of his pen against the card in front of him, he did it: "Drinking"

STOP

Video Games
Drinking

It seemed strange written down on that card, but he also felt a sensation of relief and hope sweep over him as he sat there. A sober life? He had a hard time even imagining what that would be like. But he was ready to find out. He knew that he couldn't write down "drink less" or "stop getting drunk". He felt a deep conviction about this first step, and was ready to find out what life was like without alcohol.

Still alone in the living room, his attention turned to his roommates, Derek and Chris. What would they think if they heard about these changes? They would be *pissed* about the PlayStation, that's for sure - especially Derek. And if he told them he wasn't going to be drinking anymore they might deem him crazy.

The three of them were kind of like brothers, having been friends since freshmen year. Man, they were so young, Zach recalled. So different. He remembered how Chris had come to college with very few life experiences outside of baseball and his dad's church. He had spent every Sunday listening to his own father preach as well as every Wednesday night at Youth Group. When they were freshmen, Chris had taken Zach to a couple of Athlete Fellowship meetings, but by the time first semester had ended, not even Chris was attending, because the Athlete Fellowship was on Tuesday nights -- the same night as 10-cent wings at O'Reilly's.

Derek had come to college from a totally different place than Chris, having lived with his aunt and uncle during his last year of high school, after his parents went through a nasty divorce. Zach remembered how Derek carried a silver flask to hold his liquor during that first fall together. He got the nickname "Hobo" from the upperclassmen because of it.

Nearly five years later, Zach was hit with the reality that not much had changed. The three of them were like peas in a pod, living together practically still on campus, like college had never ended.

A crazy inclination hit Zach as he read the index card, then scanned the living room of the apartment - it's time for me to move out. Maybe the #1 thing I have to "Stop" is living here, like this, with these guys. It's holding me back. *It's holding them back.*

He wrote a third step on the card: "Move out"

STOP

Video Games
Drinking
Move Out

That wasn't exactly a bad habit that he had to stop, but it felt like it fit with the assignment that Tyler had given him.

He glanced at his phone and realized it was time to get going to catch the bus to work. He got up, placed the index card in his back pocket, and headed outside.

He walked the few blocks to the bus stop, realizing that he had a few minutes to wait before the bus would arrive. His phone buzzed in his pocket, and he took it out to see the message on the screen from an unknown number:

Still have the PS4?
I'm interested in buying it

Yes. Price is firm $500.

Great. When can we meet up?
We live close to campus.

I can have it ready this afternoon
if you are able to stop over at my place.
I live close to campus too.
Cash only. Maybe 4:30?

Done. I'm Dave, by the way

Zach texted Dave his address, and that was that. Not only had he taken a step to 'stop' wasting time playing video games, but he followed it up with action, and the PS4 would be gone later that day.

A moment later the bus arrived and Zach climbed the steps, ready to grind out another day at work.

Chapter 13
Following Through

Zach arrived home that afternoon and went straight to the living room. He packaged together the PS4 with the games and controllers.

As he sat down at the couch and peered down the hallway at the box of electronics, a slight tinge of mourning came over him. Letting go of video games was like leaving a part of his childhood and teenage years behind. But he knew it was the right thing to do, the next step in his journey to becoming a better man.

He leaned forward and pulled the index card out of his pocket. He set it down on the coffee table and reviewed the three 'Stop' steps he had written down, realizing that the next two, no more drinking and moving out, would be much tougher than selling the PS4.

A moment later Derek emerged from his room, apparently having awoken from an afternoon nap, his hair disheveled, wearing just boxer shorts and a t-shirt. Passing by the living room without looking up, he shuffled into the kitchen. Zach heard the refrigerator open and the sound of Derek getting himself a can of beer.

He took a long sip as he ambled into the living room. Without even a grunt, he plopped himself down on the couch next to Zach and gazed straight ahead at the TV.

"Zach, uh, I think we've been robbed," Derek said matter-of-factly as he stared at the empty space below the TV where the PlayStation normally sat, "The PS4. It's, uh, gone."

"Yeah, I know," Zach acknowledged. He pointed to the cardboard box in the front hallway, just within their line of sight. "I sold it on Craigslist. The buyer should be here in a few minutes to pick it up."

"You WHAT?! You sold our PS4, just like that?"

"Hold on a second, Derek. It technically is, or was, *my* PS4, and I am selling what's mine. I'm trying some new things and I figured it was time to grow up a little, time to stop playing video games."

"Whatever, Zach," Derek's anger came through clearly in his tone, "You could have talked to me about it, and to Chris. What are we supposed to do now?"

"You would have only tried to talk me out of it."

Derek's irritation continued, "Is it the money? You need the cash that bad?"

"Not at all, it's nothing like that. I am trying to grow up a little."

Zach knew that Derek and Chris would be ticked, and that's what made this process difficult. He remembered Tyler's story of how difficult it was to break up with his girlfriend, even though he knew it was the right thing to do.

Derek leaned forward set his beer can down on the coffee table. His eyes caught the index card on the table. His brow furrowed as he picked it up and began to read, "What's this? STOP?"

Zach reached for the card, but Derek sprung up from the couch quickly and held the card away from Zach. Derek quickly read out loud the card's contents:

"Stop: One, Video Games. Two, Drinking. Three, Move out. What the hell is this? Is this your plan? What is going on, dude?!"

Zach's heart sank a little and he gritted his teeth, "Give me the card, Derek."

Derek spun the card out of his hand and it helicoptered to the floor, "That's it? You're gonna quit drinking and move out, like that?"

Zach was tempted to fire back at Derek, but he knew that wasn't right. He genuinely valued their friendship, and he wanted Derek to understand what was going on. He took a deep breath.

"Here's the thing. You guys are my best friends. We've got a lot of history and have had some great times. But college is over. I am not sure when you look around you see what I see. Things aren't so great. We live like we are still in school, but for me, it's time to move on."

Derek was listening, Zach could tell, so he continued.

"I have to move on to the next chapter of my life, and to do that, I have to close this one. That may corny, but it's true."

Zack picked up the index card.

"These aren't easy things. But they are what's best for me, and honestly, my moving out and moving on might be what's best for you too."

Derek sat down on the couch and sipped his beer. He shook his head.

"Hey man, you gotta do what's best for you, Zach, I get it. Truth is, you have a point."

There was a knock at the front door.

"That's my PS4 buyer, I bet," Zach said as he walked to the hallway to pick up the box of video game items.

He opened the front door to see two people standing there, an older guy and a young kid who appeared to be 12 or 13. The man stuck out his hand with a small wad of cash in it.

"It's all there," he said, handing Zach the five crisp $100 bills.

"Great, and here's all the stuff that I listed would be included," Zach replied, handing him the box.

He undid the top of it and the boy peered inside, his face excited as he anticipated taking the console and games home.

"OK, son," said the man, "you earned it." He looked at Zach, "I told him, straight A's on his report card, and he gets a PS4. Didn't think he'd do it."

With that exchange they shook hands and the man and his son returned to their still-running SUV and drove off. Zach held the $500 cash in his hand, then stuffed it into his front pocket and closed the front door.

He strode down the hallway to the living room where Derek still sat silently on the couch. Shaking his head,

Derek smiled slightly, "I have to give you credit, Zach. That PS4 was our baby. To sell it like that takes guts."

He paused and slumped into the couch cushions, "The 'new' Zach is on the horizon, huh? I guess everyone has to grow up sometime."

Zach didn't know what to say. He tapped the wad of cash in his hand. "And for me, that time is now."

Chapter 14
Step 3: SERVE

Saturday morning Zach was up early. He made himself a cup of coffee and wheat toast with butter. He threw on sweatpants and a Southern State baseball t-shirt. He grabbed his "STOP" card and put it in his pocket. Pulling his cap over his head and grabbing his baseball glove, he headed out to meet Derek at the ballfield as he had promised.

It was about a 30-minute walk to the field in a neighborhood just south of the State campus. It wasn't the roughest area of the city, but it wasn't exactly the nicest, either. As he got closer to his destination, the small houses looked to be in various states of neglect. Empty beer bottles and discarded burger wrappers littered the unkempt yards.

He arrived at the simple ballfield surrounded by a short chain-link fence. Plain wooden benches served as dugouts. Tyler was on the infield with a wide steel field dragger, pulling it behind him between first and second base. It appeared that he had dragged most of the infield dirt. Tyler looked up at Zach without stopping his task, "Hey, Zach, right on time. Can you grab the other dragger from behind the cage and help me finish this up? Still got to line the field before the kids arrive."

Zach found the other dragger and pulled it out from behind the batting cage, finding some dirt to work along the third base line. He tossed his glove down near home plate and started pulling the heavy metal device through the infield.

After a few up-and-backs, he and Tyler had completed the task and met at home plate. They placed their steel equipment next to the sturdy lock box behind the home plate batting cage.

Tyler grabbed a key from his pocket and released the padlock on the large yellow equipment lock-box, lifting the lid and setting it into the open position. He reached in and grabbed the wheeled field-liner, plus a bag of previously used white chalk. Zach held the lid of the field marker open while Tyler lifted the bag of chalk over it and poured an ample amount into the container.

"Let's get this field lined before the kids get here, and you can tell me about your 'Stop' plan," Tyler said.

He reached into the lock-box and grabbed a spool of string with a thin metal stake attached to the end of it. He handed it to Zach. They walked to home plate and Tyler chalked a simple batter's box on each side of the plate. Next they started on the task of drawing the first base line, Zach pacing out past the bag into right field as he extended the string to serve as a guide for the chalk that Tyler was about to dispense.

As he placed the field liner along the string and began to move slowly towards Zach, Tyler started right in, "So, what are you going to Stop?"

Zach had the card in his pocket, but didn't need to take it out, since he remembered his three "Stop" steps.

"Well, number one is selling my video game system, my PS4, which I already did. Number two is…"

"Wait, you sold it?" Tyler interrupted, "That's impressive."

"Yeah, Thursday, sold it for $500. My roommates weren't too happy about it."

Tyler smiled and shook his head, "Well, that's to be expected. OK, so anything else?"

"Number two, I am quitting drinking, and number three, I am moving out."

Tyler had pushed the lining cart within a few feet of Zach, and as he finished the line he paused and made eye contact with Zach. "Those are bold steps. Will you be able to follow through?"

"I hope so."

They both stared back at the chalk line that Tyler had made while Zach held the string to keep the cart on the right path.

"It might sound trite or like I am trying too hard, but these changes, Zach, they're like that chalk line we drew. First, you make a line, you make a plan; next, you work together to execute the plan. The string served as a guide, and you had to hold it in place for me to be able to push the cart and make the correct, straight line. Is it perfect? No, but it's done and done well."

Zach studied the line and he got what Tyler was saying. With his first two steps, "Sweat" and "Stop", he had not simply made a plan, but he had executed the plan. With "Stop" he felt emboldened to quit drinking and move out, mainly because he had acted on the first one, selling the PS4.

Tyler spoke again, "Have you told anyone else about your Stop plan?"

"Well, my roommate Derek found out, and he was giving me a hard time."

"Doesn't matter how he feels about it," Tyler advised. "The fact that he knows, and I know, is a big step. This word gets thrown around a lot, but the ability to make changes takes accountability. Consider that word. It simply means that you have to give an account of your actions."

They had traveled back to home plate to start on the line from home to third base. Zach stepped backwards, lining up the string between home and third base as Tyler was talking.

He continued, "You will increase your chances of *doing* your plan because others have knowledge about it. And with me, I know about it and I am *for* it. I am on your side and want to see you succeed."

Tyler read his watch, seeing that it was almost 10:30.

"The kids will be getting here in a few minutes. I usually get between 20 and 30. Last week one of the dads stayed and helped, but he has to work this morning. We'll have two stations. I will throw some BP and if you could hit some grounders on the infield that would be great. We'll rotate after 20 minutes and finish with some Tiger ball. We wrap up at 11:30."

They completed the third base line chalk and went together to the area behind the batting cage to put their equipment back into the storage box.

"You do this every Saturday?" Zach asked.

"Yep, April and May, then we try to play a few games in June. Baseball in the city is sort of a dying thing. But through the mayor's office, I have been able to secure some funding for this as a pilot project. I pulled some strings, the few that I can pull. This is only the second year, and if I can get more volunteers, I plan to expand it to other fields around the city. Most of the funding was used to fix up this field and to get gloves for the kids, a few bats, and of course the baseballs, which we lose a ton of because many of the foul balls are hit over the fence and never seen again."

Tyler pointed to the first base foul area, where a three-foot fence offered little protection from errant baseballs from rolling across the street and down the sloping hill of vacant lots.

At that moment, a skinny, pale-faced kid wearing jeans and a basketball tank-top wheeled up on his bike, his baseball glove hanging securely over one of the handlebars.

"Jeremiah!" Tyler greeted him with a smile.

"Hey coach, Jonas isn't coming today. My mom said he can't play until he gets all As and Bs, like you said." "Rules are rules, Miah," Tyler commented. "Glad you're here. You ready for some ball?"

"Yes sir," the boy replied, leaning his bike along the fence.

A couple dozen kids showed up over the next 20 minutes. Tyler gathered them at home plate, going over the rules of "respect", "effort", and "positive attitude", telling them to "REP" themselves, their families, and their community with pride.

Zach found himself totally immersed in the activities of the next hour, hitting grounders to short and second. He learned most of the kids' names in that short hour. He always seemed to have a knack for remembering names. His body worked up a good sweat. The time flew by, and before he knew it, the session was over and Tyler gathered everyone at home plate to wrap things up.

He summarized the day's baseball lessons as the ballplayers all took a knee, listening intently. He dismissed them and reminded them to shake the coaches' hands as they left. Zach stood by as the kids, one at a time, approached him, made eye contact, and gave him a solid handshake, each saying "thank you." Within minutes, he and Tyler were the only ones left at the field, and Tyler was ready to share the next step in the process of change.

He slid an index card out of his pocket and handed it to Zach, who read the single word written across the top:

SERVE

"Zach, you just experienced the third of the five steps - Serve."

"For me, this has been a real key to finding a life that is more fulfilling and meaningful. The world around us is constantly bombarding us with self-centered messages, telling us that to be happy we need to buy more, have more, eat more, etc. But true fulfillment comes when we use our lives to help others."

Zach was listening, and what Tyler's message rang true. His life throughout college was very self-focused and he couldn't think of very many situations in which he was helping or serving others. In the last hour he had experienced a unique sense of purpose and joy, one that was different from the approach of most people. Being out on that field with those kids, giving *away* to them his energy, talent, knowledge and time, he felt more *full* than empty.

Tyler continued, "After college, my dad took me with him to Honduras for a week. He's an eye doctor. We went to a rural village where I helped him give hundreds of eye exams every day, and where we handed out glasses to kids and to parents. When we weren't doing the exams, I spent most of my time there playing with the kids, mainly soccer. It was a blast. On the flight home to the States, I told my dad that I couldn't wait to go back the next year. He challenged me on that mindset. Why wait until next year? There are opportunities to serve right in front of you, every day, he said. A few months later, I started helping out as a volunteer assistant for a little league team, and that is what led me to start this."

Loading the last of the equipment into the lockbox, Zach spoke up, "To be honest, I have never really done anything like this, other than the few required community service things we had to do in college. But those seemed forced. Today didn't feel that way at all."

"I am glad to hear that. You definitely have a knack for working with kids and teaching baseball, from what I could observe."

Zach spoke up with a spontaneous but serious statement, "I already know what I am going to write on the card. I should come and help every Saturday."

Tyler's face lit up and he smiled with a chuckle, "That sounds like a great plan! Are you serious? Honestly, I was going to suggest that you write down a commitment to serve others for a minimum of one hour every week."

Zach was sure, and he knew that it was a good fit, "Absolutely. I'm sure"

"OK, that's your Serve."

"What's else? I mean, is there another step?" Zach felt like he was on a roll with these changes and didn't want to let the momentum slow.

"There are two more steps. Tomorrow, meet me at the Downtown Farmer's Market at 2 pm, and we'll get going with number four." Tyler instructed, "But, more importantly, remind yourself of steps one and two and keep working at them. Be accountable to me and to yourself for those steps. Do I have your permission to ask you if you are moving forward with your Sweat and Stop steps?"

Zach was ready. He knew that since it was a typical Saturday night, he would face his roommates and have to tell Chris that he was giving up drinking and planning to move out, if Derek hadn't told him already.

"Yes, I would appreciate that."

"You got it."

Zach grabbed his glove from the dirt, gave it a couple smacks to get the dust off, and they shook hands. "See you tomorrow."

Chapter 15

Searching

Zach arrived at his apartment as Chris was coming out the front door.

Chris began, "Derek tells me that you are growing up, getting sober and moving out. You gonna become a priest or something?"

Zach could hear the sarcasm in his voice. "Not exactly, but I am making some changes. It's time, man."

What Chris said next surprised Zach, "You aren't the only one. I've been meaning to tell you guys for a while...I am moving back home with my parents. My days at State are over. My dad has a friend who has been searching for someone to hire for Inside Sales, and he is willing to give me a chance. It doesn't pay much at first, but I will be living at home to save money. I start June 1st."

Zach was stunned, but also relieved. "That's great. The preacher's kid can go home after all, huh?"

They both laughed. "Yeah, I guess," said Chris.

"What about Derek?" Zach realized.

Chris made his way down the steps in front of the apartment and onto the curb, clicking his key to unlock the door to his truck. "It will be good for him. We all have to move on eventually, right?"

Chris hopped in his truck and pulled away, leaving Zach standing outside the apartment. It occurred to him that perhaps more was going on with Chris than he had cared to appreciate or ask about. *I am not the only one*, he thought.

That Saturday night Zach made a bold decision to stay in and stay sober. He knew it wouldn't be easy but yet he knew it was right. He thought about going out but also considered what it would be like to stay true to his promise to stick to his plan.

He spent the night hunting online for apartments, something that he could afford; simple places not as close to the campus as where he currently lived. There were several available not far from the ballfield where he and Tyler had run the clinic that morning. He inquired about a couple that looked promising, sending emails to the landlords. Most were one bedroom flats, simple but also perfect for this new stage of his life.

He found himself bored though content. It occurred to him around 10 or 11 p.m. that it might have been the first Saturday night that he was sober for many months. It was refreshing. He felt clear minded, alive and somewhat renewed. He could sense this chapter of his life coming to a close as if he was turning a page in a book. He was anxious to learn steps number four and five in Tyler's plan. As he lay awake in bed that night he started to reminisce about college: the thrills on the baseball field, the moments of genuine friendship between Derek and Chris and him, the road trips, the struggle of early morning practices. College had been an amazing experience. He acknowledged a tinge of sadness as he knew that there was no turning back, but also felt hope arise as he considered the possibility of a new amazing waiting for him if he chose to take the right steps. Eventually he drifted off to sleep.

Chapter 16
Sunday Morning

Without an alarm, Zach was up by 8:30 the next morning. There hadn't been many Sunday mornings that he remembered being up before noon and he found himself kind of bored. Sitting in his room and looking at more apartments online, it occurred to him that he had time to go and see a few of them, at least from the outside. His focus was almost solely on places close to the ballfield where he'd been the morning before. They were affordable, and it was far enough away from campus that he would find himself separate from the college atmosphere. He decided to take a run and investigate the area.

A bonus run? After one round of running three mornings a week to work, he felt he was starting to get into shape. He didn't exactly feel *athletic* or *fit*, but he was better off than a couple of weeks ago.

He put on his shoes, a pair of old shorts, and a T-shirt. He took out his phone and viewed the map of the area where most of the apartments he was considering were located - only 1.3 miles away. He decided he could manage a 2.5 to 3-mile loop.

As he ran that morning, he had time to reflect about the last couple weeks of his life. He pondered the changes he was making - he'd decided to Sweat in order to rediscover the athletic core that was a big part of who he was, he had taken steps to Stop in three areas of his life that were holding him back. He had committed to Serve each week with Tyler through the baseball program. They were all positive steps, but they weren't easy. His mind was filled with a mixture of relief, excitement, and a bit of a fear of the unknown. His old life had provided security in his set ways, and these changes were unsettling even if they were positive.

His pace slowed as he turned that corner where some of the apartments were. He sadly surveyed one of the buildings. The listing online had made it seem pretty nice, but at close range it was very rundown.

He continued past the ballfield where he and Tyler worked with the kids. He paused and examined the field, the vacant lots and sloping hill behind the first base fence. He remembered Tyler mentioning how many baseballs got lost when foul balls were hit over that fence. Zach studied the home-plate backstop, a small and not-so-sturdy metal structure. He considered the possible solutions to all those lost baseballs. A bigger backstop? A taller fence? Perhaps a tall attachment of netting to prevent balls from flying over?

He remembered Tyler had secured only a small grant from the mayor's office to pilot the program. He imagined that the cost of some netting attached to the top of the fence would be around $500. He remembered the $500 cash he had sitting in his room from selling the PS4. *Maybe I should check on the price of improving this part of the baseball field*, he thought.

He continued, rounding the block on the opposite side of the field, then turning to go a little further away from campus. This area was somewhat depressed, but he observed a mixture of well-cared-for properties and some that were clearly neglected. There were three and four story apartment buildings as well as a few rows of single family homes, many with detached one-car garages behind their narrow driveways.

As he headed down a side street, he noticed a small, simple house with a sign in the front yard "Apartment for

Rent." He didn't recognize it from anything he had seen online, and the sign didn't list a phone number. He stopped to take a closer look. The house was small but well-kept. He guessed only a couple of bedrooms, probably 1,000 square feet. Where was the apartment? He took a couple more steps and glanced down the driveway to see a detached garage, and above it a second story with wooden steps leading up the side. He surveyed the area. It was quiet, and the majority of the properties on this block were well-maintained, with small grass front yards, clean landscaping, and covered front porches.

Zach heard a voice from behind him, "Can I help you?" It was an older women's voice, he could tell, like a grandma's.

A short, thin lady stood on the porch of the house wearing jeans and a sweatshirt, her face framed by old-school glasses. She had a ball cap on over her black hair, which was pulled back into a ponytail.

Zach spoke up, "Oh hi, sorry. I was in the area and noticed your sign for the apartment. Is it still available?"

"It is. Are you interested?" she said as she walked the short distance to meet him.

"Yes, ma'am," He said confidently as he reached out his hand with a smile, "I'm Zach."

She shook his hand in return, "I'm Meredith Smith. Would you like to take a look?"

"If that's alright with you, I mean, I don't want to be a bother."

"It's no bother, son," she said as they strolled up the driveway. "It's a lovely place, not big, but clean. And you have your own kitchen, so you won't have much to worry about."

They climbed the steps. She took a set of keys from her pocket, unlocking the wooden door as they stood on the platform at the top of the steps.

She motioned for Zach to go on ahead as she continued, "Before my husband passed he had this place renovated as a way to bring income in after he retired. It's been a steady flow ever since, but our last renter took a job in Atlanta, so it's up to me to find a new one. My husband handled all the renters in the past, and I have been kind of slow about getting someone new in here."

Zach assessed the simple, studio-style apartment. It was an open floor plan, with a well-equipped kitchen, a cozy living room, and a dining area that could probably fit a table for four.

"I am sorry for your loss ma'am, I mean, of your husband."

"Thirty-nine years, we were married. He was a good man, and took care of me like a husband should." She walked ahead of Zach, "Here is the only bedroom, and there is the bathroom." She pointed to left of where they were standing. Zach went ahead of her down a narrow hallway, opening the door to a clean, updated bathroom.

"What do you think?" she asked.

"It's great. It's exactly what I am looking for."

They returned to the main room. She picked up a couple of papers from the kitchen counter.

"Like I said, Frank handled all of this before he passed. These papers are the next step. You can see there the lease agreement, and the conduct agreement. Frank added that one on his own. Said it would weed out the bad ones."

She handed Zach the papers. "I bet you are wondering about the price, right? Well, here's the thing," she went on. "It's $500 a month, but I have been considering giving a little bit of a discount if I can find someone to help me with the yard. Frank did that too, and with my arthritis, the mowing and weeding are too much."

"Ma'am, that price is more than fair and I would be happy to help with the yard, no discount needed," Zach asserted.

"That's awfully kind of you. When were you hoping to move in?" She was eager to close the deal.

They headed outside, down the steps, and up the driveway to the front of the house.

"Wow. Can I take a day to think about it?"

"Sure you can, Zach. But how about in good faith I do this," she leaned down and pulled the 'Apartment for Rent' sign from its spot in the front grass, "I'll take this inside. Why don't you stop by tomorrow and let me know."

"I'll do that," Zach agreed as they shook hands.

"Bye-bye now," she said with a kind smile.

"See you tomorrow," he promised as he slowly started his jog home.

Chapter 17
Step 4: SUSTENANCE

That afternoon, Zach took the bus downtown, arriving at the outdoor green space where the weekly Farmers Market took place. He'd never been to it before, and he was surprised at the large crowd of people and dozens of vendors selling fresh produce and a wide variety of other goods.

He got there a little before 2 o'clock and spotted Tyler right away standing in the distance. He was holding a couple of empty canvas bags and leaning against a bike rack.

They greeted each other and began to visit the rows of produce booths.

Tyler spoke up, "I bet you are eager for number four on the list, huh?"

"Yes I am, but I have some news to tell you about first. I may have found a new place to live. It's a one-bedroom and it's a block from the ballfield."

"That's great. Man, you are indeed a person of action, Zach. And the price?"

"Right in the range I was hoping for. I will be able to save some money, and it's private, above a garage over on Devonshire Street."

Tyler nodded. "That's a good spot, Zach. Quiet area. Most of those people have lived there for a long time. You might be the youngest person on the street!"

They continued to stroll among the vendors, with Tyler purchasing a variety of fresh fruits and vegetables. As they came to the end of the row, Tyler led the way to a bench, where they sat down, facing the busy market.

Tyler reached into his pocket and pulled out the next index card, handing it to Zach.

SUSTENANCE

Zach looked down at the word quizzically.

Tyler began, "A strange one, huh? You may have noticed that the first three steps were verbs, and this is a noun. Obviously, I have tried to find words that *best* describe the essence of how I try to live. I toyed with the word 'sustain' but it didn't have the same ring of truth. 'Sustain' sounds static, while 'Sustenance' is the best way to describe this step. There are things that you need to eliminate from your life. Those were the Stops, which you are doing a great job with. But we also need to feed our lives with good things. This word is the most literal of the steps. Do you know the dictionary definition of 'sustenance'?" Tyler asked.

"Not really. Makes me think of food."

"Exactly," confirmed Tyler, taking an apple out of one of his bags, "I've got the definition memorized, and here is it: *food and drink regarded as a source of strength; nourishment.* Pretty simple. Right?"

"Yes, yes it is." Zach acknowledged.

Tyler reached into the bag and pulled out a bell pepper.

"These are couple of my go-to's. Fruits and vegetables. As a kid, I hated anything these didn't contain the words 'peanut butter and jelly' but I have grown to thoroughly enjoy eating a wide variety of healthy, real food."

Zach sat back, mulling over his diet. He survived college on pizza, beer, and well, more pizza and more beer. He glanced down at his gut, not proud of the potbelly shape.

119

Tyler put the produce back into the bag and continued, "My mantra is 'good stuff in, good life out, garbage in, garbage out'. I consistently make an effort to eat healthy. I have more energy. I'm 32, but I feel better than I did 10 years ago." He sat up straight and handed the card to Zach, rotating towards him as they sat on the bench.

"Don't get me wrong. I am not some kind of super-strict dieter. I still have the occasional burger or bags of chips, and my Achilles' heel is still Reese's Peanut Butter Cups!"

Zach sighed deeply. He'd never given much consideration to what he ate. As a young college athlete, he had a strong, lean body. But in one year beyond baseball, his body had changed dramatically. He knew that this next step was what he needed, but it wasn't anything to get excited about. He was honest with Tyler, "I don't know about this one, Tyler, this 'sustenance.' I'm trying to eat cheap and fast most of the time."

"This step is a struggle. That's why it's number four. Take a risk. Try it. Start simple. Here is what I want you to do with that card. Write down five, just five, healthy foods or drinks that you will try to consume regularly. They can be simple, like water or a banana or an apple. Try it for a week."

Zach realized that what Tyler was asking was manageable. It wasn't a total diet takeover, merely a few simple changes.

"I suppose I can manage that."

"Great," Tyler encouraged him, "and I believe that you can do it."

They stood up from the bench.

"My bike's locked up on the rack down at the other end." Tyler informed him.

"OK, cool. I am going to catch the bus here," Zach said, motioning towards the corner close to where they were sitting.

"The fifth and final step - you wondering about that?" asked Tyler.

"Yes, you bet."

"OK, this one is a little bit of a bonus step, one that some people are up for and others take a pass on, so promise me that you will keep an open mind."

Zach was ready for anything at this point, "So far, so good. I'm up for whatever."

"Love the positive attitude, Zach. It's a men's group. We meet every Friday morning at 5:45 am in the basement of St. John's Church downtown, right next to the courthouse."

"A men's group?" Zach asked, "Like Freemasons or something?"

"No, it's more of a spiritual thing. Like I said, it's not for everyone. Technically, you might call it a Bible Study, but there are lots of guys there from various walks of life and backgrounds."

Zach could feel his body language change as he became hesitant and nervous. He had not really been to anything like what Tyler was talking about, and he pictured in his mind a bunch of guys holding hands and singing church hymns.

"Listen, I understand, it's different from the other steps, but I have to be my authentic, real self if I am going to share with you what has changed my life, and this group has been a big part of that. It would be insincere of me *not* to invite you." Tyler was speaking calmly, but with bold seriousness.

"That sounds fair. I don't have to join or anything if I go this one time, right?" Zach said.

"Of course not," Tyler assured him.

"Alright, I will come on Friday. And by then I will have lost 10 pounds from eating all fruits and veggies!" Zach joked.

"Just five. Five items you'll make a regular part of what you eat." Tyler and Zach shook hands.

As Zach walked across the street to the bus stop, he realized that step five wasn't a big deal. He'd never had much 'spiritual' input into his life, and maybe a 'guy group' would be a good change. Besides, if it was in the city, he could make some connections with men who could help him get out of his dead-end job and into something better. *It's a new chapter in my life,* he thought, *yet I still have a job that I don't like.*

As he considered his week ahead, he looked forward to the exercise he would get, to trying to change some of what he was eating, and even to finalizing the deal on the new apartment. But one thing he wasn't looking forward to was five days of road crew work with the City Maintenance department. After all, he had a Marketing degree. He'd take a pay cut to work in some kind of job where he was putting his skills and education to good use. It wasn't that he didn't value the ability to work and earn a living. He knew that this job had been one that gave him the dignity that comes with hard work. But he also yearned to have his work be more in line with his gifts, experiences, and passion. He decided to start searching for an opportunity, even an internship, where he would do just that.

The bus arrived and he climbed aboard for the 20-minute ride to his apartment.

Chapter 18
Sustenance Steps

Monday morning Zach got up a little earlier than he needed to, and before getting ready for his run to work, he sat down at the kitchen table with his "Sustenance" card to write down his list of five items. The first one was easy:

"Water" he wrote down, "at least 60 ounces a day"

He paused for a moment. He knew that bananas were a good source of nutrition, and relatively cheap.

"4 bananas per week"

He thought about vegetables. He wasn't a big fan. But he could stomach a salad every once in a while.

"1 salad for lunch each week"

Three down, two to go. He figured he'd better put an item on the list that had some real calories.

"Lean protein: Fish, grilled chicken, or a protein bar. Every day."

That was a good step, and he could easily buy a box of protein bars as a go-to snack.

One more item. He recalled a trip that he'd taken with his family out west as a kid. His dad had packed a bag of Trail Mix for him and his younger sister. He remembered that it was pretty good - it had peanuts, raisins, granola, and a small amount of chocolate chips. He knew that he could manage to make some of that and it would be a good way to snack on something healthy. He wrote it down, "Trail Mix"

There it was, his five items for Sustenance:

SUSTENANCE

Water – at least 60 ounces a day

4 Bananas per week

1 Salad for lunch each week

Lean protein: Fish, grilled chicken, or a protein bar. Every day.

Trail Mix

He put the card in his pocket, and remembered his promise to Meredith to stop by and finalize the lease on the apartment. He planned to do that right after work. As he surveyed at his belongings in his room, he realized that moving would be pretty easy. He didn't own much; his bed, his dresser and desk, and one of the couches in the living room. The rest of the apartment furniture was either Derek's or Chris'.

He stepped outside, the April sun shining down through the trees as he began his run to work.

Chapter 19
Signed

"Hey, Zach, come on in!" Mrs. Smith called after hearing his knock on the front door.

He stepped inside the modest living room, simply decorated, and immediately noticed the row of framed family pictures above the floral-print couch. She led him through the room into the small kitchen, where she had the lease papers side-by-side on the two-person table.

"Are you ready to sign on the dotted line?" she quizzed.

"Yes, ma'am." Zach smiled, pulling out one of the chairs to sit.

"Take your time and read through it all. The conduct agreement is brief but thorough. Frank had it down to a science," she said confidently.

Zach read over the documents.

"As you can see, rather than first and last month's rent, he asked for a $200 deposit. He said that people today operated on distrust, and his way, a smaller up-front amount, built trust. We've had three different renters over these last few years, and not once has anyone been late on rent." She shook her head in admiration of her late husband, "Frank was a good man...a good man."

"That sure is a different way of doing things," Zach agreed as he finished signing the papers, standing up from the table to reach into his pocket. He pulled out two $100 bills from his wallet and placed them on the table, "and I won't break that trust, Mrs. Smith."

"Oh, dear, please call me Meredith," she chuckled as they walked towards the front door. "Let's see, today's the 16th, so I will see you back here on the 29th or 30th to move in?"

"Yes, ma'am, that sounds good to me," he confirmed, stepping out through the front door and pivoting to shake her hand.

"Great, Zach. I'm glad that this worked out so quickly."

"So am I, Mrs. Sm.., I mean Meredith," he said with a tip of his ball cap.

On the walk home he realized he had the rest of the week to keep working on his "S" plan, since he wouldn't see Tyler until the men's group on Friday at 5:45 am. He felt like it was a good amount of time to really focus in - especially on Sweat and Sustenance - and also to keep his commitment to Stop.

On his way home he took a slight detour and zipped into a local grocery store that had a large organic foods section. He picked up a bundle of bananas, ingredients needed to make his trail mix, a box of protein bars, and a package of lean chicken breasts. The girl at the checkout reviewed his purchases and he could tell that she was quite impressed with his healthy choices. Holding a brown paper grocery bag in each arm, he went the rest of the way home.

That week Zach was determined to keep making progress, working hard to exercise, eat right, and stay solid in his commitment to Stop. He was up early each morning, ate a banana and some oatmeal to start his day, and was able to make his jog to work at a slightly quicker pace.

At home, he spent most of his time packing boxes in his room, sorting through many old items from college; clothes, books, notebooks, and more Southern State baseball swag than he could believe. He filled three large garbage bags that he planned to donate to Goodwill.

On Wednesday morning, he got a text from Tyler.

Just checking in. Hope you are working your plan to the fullest!

Yes I am! See you early on Friday!

Zach was once again reminded of one *major* area in his life where things weren't lined up exactly as he would hope: his job. He had started to look online for marketing internships, but many of the job qualifications mentioned "experience" as a requirement.

It occurred to him that maybe he should pursue a job working with kids, as his day helping Tyler at the baseball program was so enjoyable. He knew that community centers in the area didn't have many available positions. He decided that he would talk to Tyler about it when he saw him on Friday. Maybe he would have some wisdom to share.

Chapter 20
Step 5: SEEK

Friday morning Zach's alarm rang at 5:20 am., waking him from a sound sleep. He rose slowly, putting on his running clothes, sliding a pair of sweatpants over his shorts and a hoodie over his t-shirt. Tyler assured him that "church clothes" were not required and that the men's group was "come as you are." He grabbed a banana and headed outside for the short hike to the bus stop.

He took a different bus than normal, and gazed out the window at the houses and buildings. A faint light began to emerge as the sun rose on the horizon.

Tyler let him know that he would have an extra Bible for him, and Zach was relieved since he didn't own one and hadn't seen one outside of a church pew since he was a little kid.

As his bus arrived on the corner across the street from St. John's, he saw several middle-aged men walking in the through a propped-open side door, each carrying a coffee in one hand with a Bible in the other. He had neither, and suddenly he felt a bit nervous. For a moment, he was tempted to bail out and began to consider an excuse that would be believable to Tyler.

At that moment he saw Tyler get out of his parked car, holding the two Bibles. He realized that he had better follow through on his promise to attend, even if it was this one time. Tyler had done a lot for him, and it didn't feel right to bail.

He departed the bus and marched across the street.

"Zach, up bright and early!"

"You can say that again. It's been a while since I was up before the sun. Probably college, for fall conditioning." Zach remembered his least favorite part of being a baseball player.

"Thankfully, we'll be sitting, not running, for about the next hour," Tyler said. "Remember, keep an open mind. These guys may surprise you."

At the church, they went down a few steps into the basement. To Zach it had that distinct "church" smell, a little stale, with the scent of bad coffee in the air.

In a large room, seven or eight rows of metal chairs faced a small podium on the left wall. On the far end of the room was a kitchen with a pass-through counter. Sitting on top of it were two tall coffee containers. Some men stood and talked while others sat in the rows of chairs, keeping to themselves. As his eyes scanned the room, Zach guessed that most of the 35 or 40 guys were in their 40s or 50s, some dressed for business, while others wore jeans, work shirts, and baseball caps. There were a couple of senior-citizen-looking men, and the group was a mixture of white men and a few black men.

Tyler handed Zach the extra Bible he had brought with him, "Here you go."

They found their way to a couple of seats near the back and Zach settled in, placing his Bible on his lap. A moment later, a tall black man with glasses and a shiny bald head stood at the podium.

"Good morning, men!" He commanded them with a booming voice, "If everyone could have their seats, we can get this thing going."

The men who had been standing took their seats and became attentive and quiet as Rick continued.

"Welcome to Week #965 of the Friday morning men's group! That's right, we are halfway through our 18th year of meeting right here in the basement of St. John's. Are there any new guys here this morning? Please stand and introduce yourself to the rest of us. C'mon, be bold."

Tyler gave Zach a slight elbow jab. Zach slowly rose to his feet. A man a row in front of him and to his right stood, as did an older guy in the front row.

"Let's start up here. Tell us about yourself," Rick said, making eye contact with a man up in the front.

"Well, my name in Henry Dietrich, and I'm retired. I worked as an administrator at the University for 29 years. I came here today with my good friend Dale Whitlock."

"Great, Henry, we are glad to have you," Rick motioned towards Zach. "And you, young man."

Zach spoke nervously as all of the heads in the room turned to listen. "My name is Zach Welton, and I work for the city. I just graduated, well, I mean, I graduated last year from State. And Tyler brought me."

Rick replied to Zach's introduction, "Tyler is at it again. Zach, you probably wouldn't be surprised to hear that there are probably 10 or 12 guys here today who were first invited by Tyler."

"No sir, that wouldn't surprise me at all," Zach confirmed.

"Welcome, Zach, we are glad to have someone so young among us! It definitely ups the 'cool' quotient of the group, right guys?" Rick commented, hearing a couple of muted chuckles.

Zach sat down, sighing and feeling a bit relieved as all eyes returned to the front of the room. It was a lot like Tyler had described; a bunch of normal guys, and the atmosphere was relaxed. After the final new person was introduced, Rick transitioned. "Men, we again this week have the privilege of receiving the teaching wisdom of Dr. David Riggins, our long time leader. Dr. Dave has been leading us through a series on the book of Galatians. Dr. Dave…"

A solidly-built man stood up from the front row, dressed in jeans and a tucked-in flannel button-down shirt. He carried with him a leather Bible and plain notebook.

"Thank you, Rick, and welcome, good men, and especially our new men," he said in a confident, smooth tone, making brief eye contact in turn with Zach and the other first-timers. He placed his belongings on the podium and continued. "Men, if you would turn in your Bibles to Galatians 2, the first verse, that is where we left off last week," he requested.

Zach flipped open his Bible, trying to sneak a peek at Tyler's to see exactly where in the Bible Galatians was. He noticed Tyler leafing through the pages to almost the end of the book, so he scanned the top of the pages until he found the right spot, thumbing through until he saw the heading "Chapter 2."

Dr. Dave began by reading out loud a paragraph from the text. He reminded the audience of the context, the previous week's lessons and how they connected, and the relevance of the passage for their lives today. Some men took detailed notes while others simply listened. Zach could tell that Dr. Dave was intelligent and knew the content well. He was an engaging and commanded the attention of everyone in the room. Zach didn't understand some of what was talked about, but there was a ring of truth to the overall teaching.

The time flew by and Dr. Dave concluded his time with a brief prayer. All of the men said "Amen" in unison, and the room was again filled with conversation as they each made their way out at their own pace.

Zach and Tyler walked out together, the city streets more crowded with early morning commuters and a bit of traffic. He handed Tyler back the borrowed Bible.

"What did you think?" Tyler asked right away, handing Zach an index card that he had been keeping in between the pages of his Bible.

"It was interesting. Different than what I expected."

Zach saw on the card the last of the five "S" steps that Tyler had been leading him through:

SEEK

"Yes, that's usually what I hear. Most guys assume it's gonna be some kind of cult or weird thing where guys are singing or being drilled with Bible quiz questions," Tyler commented as they moved toward his parked car.

"Exactly. I was nervous that I was going to feel like an outsider and people would judge me for not knowing certain church stuff."

"Right. Dr. Dave has a way of putting people at ease. He was a fighter pilot in the Navy and served in the first Gulf War. He's also been the President of Second National Bank, and now he manages a foundation that gives grants to nonprofits. The guy is impressive."

"Impressive. And he seems to know his Bible pretty well, too," Zach said.

"He does. And for me, his teachings have given me insight into myself, the world around me, and my place in it. That's why it says 'Seek' on that card. It doesn't say Bible Study or God or church. It says seek. Seek truth, seek goodness, seek for a better way." Tyler was giving another speech, but Zach didn't mind. He paused, seeming to expect Zach to respond.

"Well, I've never been into the Bible or church or anything like that. But this morning was pretty cool. I'd come back." Zach said as they got closer to Tyler's car.

"Awesome. Over time you'll figure out what fits for you. Some guys, they find their place in a church and it becomes a key part of their life. I have talked with a few who are more comfortable attending this group, or just reading spiritual books. The important aspect is that you find a source of wisdom and truth that can keep you grounded and can complement the other four steps."

"That sounds very doable," Zach responded. He respected what Tyler said because he had learned to respect *who Tyler was.*

Tyler reached into his pocket and took out his keys, pushing a button to unlock his car door. He went around to the driver's side and opened it.

"That's it?" Zach asked, "The five steps are over?"

"Tomorrow morning, you are coming to the baseball clinic, right?" Tyler asked.

"I'll be there."

"Bring all five of your index cards. We'll talk a bit more then. And I have one last thing to ask you about." Tyler slid into his car and turned the key, leaving Zach on the curb to wonder what the "one last thing" was.

Zach stood for a moment, then realized that he had a nice long run ahead of him, and beyond that another long day at work. At least it was a Friday.

Chapter 21

New Beginnings

The next Saturday morning, Zach got up and ate his ritual banana and oatmeal. He grabbed his baseball glove and his five index cards. Since Tyler hadn't instructed him to do otherwise, he had left the "Seek" card blank.

He tucked them into his shorts pocket and headed outside for the long walk to the field. He took a little detour to pass by his new apartment and found Meredith on her front porch.

"Hey, Zach, where are you headed this morning, to play some ball?" She said, noticing the glove under his arm.

"No ma'am, not exactly. I am helping a friend with a youth baseball program over at the ballfield."

"Well, isn't that nice of you."

"Oh, it's a fun time. They are good kids and I have a blast teaching them the game."

"Did you play baseball as a kid?" she asked.

"Yes, ma'am, and I played here at Southern State."

"Well how about that, you must've been excellent," she said with a smile.

"I was OK, I guess."

"Have fun. Enjoy this sunny Saturday."

They concluded their little chat and he continued up the street. He realized that in a couple of weeks, it would be a very short distance from his apartment to the field, and he might even get an opportunity to get acquainted with some of the kids in the neighborhood.

He arrived at the field. It was already fully prepped. The infield was dragged and the lines chalked. Tyler sat on an upside-down plastic bucket near the third base fence, taking a sip from a water bottle.

"Tyler, you did all this without me?"

"It wasn't any hassle. I was up and got here early, so I got to work." He glanced down at his phone, "We've got 15 minutes until the kids arrive. Did you bring your five index cards?"

"Yes, I sure did," Zach reached into his pocket and pulled out the cards, handing them to Tyler.

Tyler read each to himself, filing them one at a time behind each other as he reviewed their contents.

"Zach, I have to say, these are great. Not only what you committed to change, but how you've taken action. There have been a handful of guys that I have shared these with over the years, and I have say, you have impressed me."

"Thanks. It's been a great couple of weeks. I feel like I've begun a new chapter in my life. It took me more than a year to realize it, but college, it's over. Up until this past month, if you would have asked me who I was, I probably would have said 'a college baseball player.' But those days were a long time ago. It's as if I'm starting to learn a new identity, and a new way of living and finding meaning." Zach's impromptu speech came out all at once, like a flood gate opening.

"Zach, I'm thrilled to hear that," Tyler remarked, handing him the index cards, "I'm in your corner. If it's OK with you, let's touch base every Saturday morning here at the field and talk about those cards."

"I can do that." Zach was ready to follow through fully on his commitments.

"And you are probably wondering about the surprise." Tyler grinned as he stood up from his bucket seat, "I'll be right back. It's in my car."

He walked around the fence to his parked car, and returned a moment later with a simple folder. He opened it and took out a single piece of paper that was inside of it.

"I have been working on a proposal over at the mayor's office, and I wanted you to be the first to see it."

He handed Zach the paper. Across the top of it was the mayor's office letterhead, and below that, in bold letters:

COMMUNITY OUTREACH
MARKETING AND PUBLICITY INTERNSHIP

Tyler spoke as Zach read the heading and started scanning the one-page Proposal and Job Description, "This is something that I have been working on for a couple of years, but last week I finally got it approved as an add-on to this year's PR programming budget. It's a 12-month internship. It pays, but not much. Its focus is on programs like this baseball program; building bridges in the community, raising awareness of the challenges that kids in the city are facing, and the city's overall effort to partner with the private sector and non-profits to help kids."

Tyler sounded like an expert pitchman and, as Zach reviewed the document, he saw that it would give him experience in both marketing and in working with kids in the community.

"Are you offering this to me?" Zach boldly asked.

"You are the only person I have shown it to. Since it's an internship and it's a publicly funded program, we have to post it publicly. But I'm the one doing the hiring. You'd be working directly for me." Tyler seemed excited at the idea.

"I'm honored that you would think of me. Are you sure?" Zach didn't want to overstep his assumptions about this opportunity.

"Zach, I can sense that it's a great fit. Consider it and let me know." Tyler grabbed the bucket of baseballs, carrying it to the edge of the home plate area.

Zach took the paper and folder and set it down under his glove near the fence, looking up to see Jeremiah arriving on his bike, with a smaller kid riding behind him while standing on the bike-tire pegs.

"Jeremiah!" Zach shouted warmly, "And you must be Jonas!"

"Hey Coach Zach," Jeremiah greeted back, "Yeah, this is my little bro. Jonas, this is Coach Zach, who I was telling you about."

Jonas hopped off the pegs and approached Zach, sticking out his little hand for a firm handshake. "Hi, Coach, I'm Jonas, and I am the best nine-year-old baseball player you've ever met."

"Is that so?" Zach replied. "Well, it's an honor to meet you. Remind me to get your autograph later!"

"It's a beautiful day for some baseball, Coach Zach!" Jeremiah said as he glanced up at the clear blue sky.

"Yes it is, Jeremiah. It certainly is."

Indeed, it was a beautiful new day. Zach paused and thought back over the past few weeks, and a smile came across his face. Here he was, turning the page into a new chapter of his life. He was committed to change and to becoming a person of purpose and passion. The path forward wasn't smooth or straight, but it was clear and he was determined more than ever to take step after step on his way to a truly meaningful way of life.

Questions for Reflection
or Discussion

After reading chapters 1 to 7, answer these questions:

Do you relate at all to Zach's story and where he is in his life?

Zach is experiencing somewhat of an identity crisis. If he were to fill in the blank in this scenario, what would he write? "Zach Welton, _____"

How about you? What one or two words would you use to describe your current identity?

Zach goes from struggling to finding himself at a crossroads, having blacked out after a night of binge drinking. Can you relate to this experience?

When you are alone and have time to reflect upon your life, are you at peace or do you desire change? If you are stirred to make changes, what areas are most pressing?

Step 1: SWEAT

"I looked back at my childhood, at my teenage years, and college, and all the way through I noticed that I felt most *myself* during times when I was active"
– Tyler

As you look back over your life so far, do you resonate with the statement above? If so, write down the physical activities that you have found to be most fulfilling:

Give yourself of a 'overall fitness grade' on a scale of 1 to 10:

Three years ago:
One year ago:
Today:

If you are like Zach and trying to make a change in this area, use an index card to write down your "Sweat Plan", Remember to make your plan simple, specific and smart.

Step 2: STOP

"Stop means stop. It means to take stock of your life and decide to cut out things that are holding you back." - Tyler

The world hates a quitter. But we all have areas of our life that we know are holding us back from reaching our potential. They can be bad habits or even addictions. In these areas, quitting is the best choice.

If you are like Zach and desire to make a change in this area, write down your "Stop Plan" on an index card. Remember to make your plan <u>simple</u>, <u>specific</u> and <u>smart</u>.

Following Through:

Zach's chances of success for these changes in his life increase because he has someone who is holding him accountable. Write down the name or names of one or two people who you can enlist to share this plan with who can do the same for you:

Step 3: SERVE

"The world around us is constantly bombarding us with self-centered messages, telling us that to be happy we need to buy more, have more, eat more, etc. But true fulfillment comes when we use our lives to help others." – Tyler

Write down the times in your life when you have taken your time, talents, or resources to intentionally help others.

When we only serve others through an annual trip or day of community service, the impact is limited, both for those being helped and for those doing the helping. Look around your community. What opportunities are there that you would be a good fit for?

Use an index card to write down your "Serve Plan", or write it down on an index card. Remember to make your plan <u>simple,</u> <u>specific</u> and <u>smart</u>.

Step 4: SUSTENANCE

"I've got the definition memorized: *food and drink regarded as a source of strength; nourishment.*"
- Tyler

Get a piece of paper and make a list of everything that you ate and drank in the past 48 hours.

Does that list reflect food and drink "regarded as a source of strength"? Circle anything that is helping you stay healthy.

Use an index card to write down your "Sustenance Plan", Remember to make your plan <u>simple</u>, <u>specific</u> and <u>smart</u>.

Step 5: SEEK

"Find a course of wisdom and truth that can keep you grounded and can complement the other four steps."
- Tyler

What does "seek" mean to you? Why is this the final step?

Tyler told Zach that he has found the men's group and his church to be a place of wisdom and truth. What experiences have you had in your life up until now in this area?

Use an index card to write down your "Seek Plan", Remember to make your plan <u>simple</u>, <u>specific</u> and <u>smart</u>.

More Questions for Reflection

What are the barriers preventing us from making changes, or "stopping" things in our lives?

Have you ever had moments when you knew your life needed a change? Did you act on it? Why or why not?

What are ways to combat apathy? Or to kick start motivation for change?

What is the most important step, for you, of the five steps? Or are they all equally important?

Why does Tyler have Zach focus on Sweat as the first step? Is this random, or is there something more to it?

Is there a purpose for the order of the steps?

What qualities make Tyler a good mentor?

What qualities make Zach able to benefit from the steps?

"After The Lights" Seminar

Based on content from the book, this **60 to 90-minute session** fits perfectly into the programming calendar for any NCAA athletic department and is designed to **enhance the Life Skills experience for seniors and graduate students.**

In an interactive and engaging hour to hour-and-a-half, Mark guides students through the process of getting ready for **personal fulfillment** in the next season of life.

The focus of the seminar looks beyond professional "success", helping these college athletes discover five simple steps to **find meaning** *after the lights.*

Call or Email Mark to find out more about bringing the seminar to your school.

412.865.9015
msteffey@ccojubilee.org
t: @mark_steffey
www.afterthelightsbook.com

43029467R00089

Made in the USA
Middletown, DE
28 April 2017